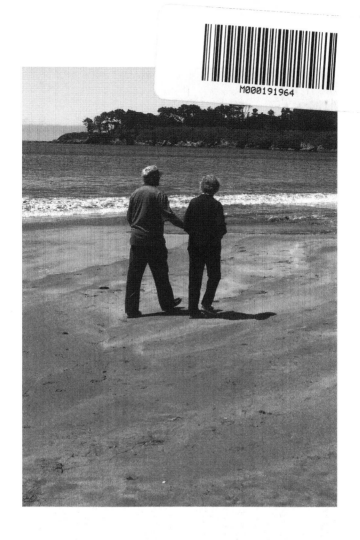

LIFELINES: A CARE
PARTNER'S SURVIVAL
GUIDE

BY

ROGER E. RILEY

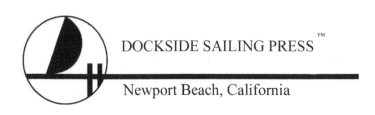

DOCKSIDE SAILING PRESS ™

Newport Beach, California

www.docksidesailingpress.com

Copyright 2014 by Roger E. Riley

P3

Printed in the United States of America

iii

DEDICATION

This book is dedicated first to my loving wife Marilyn and secondly to those individuals throughout the world whose compassion and self-sacrifice bring comfort to others suffering from Alzheimer's and other debilitating diseases needing care partners.

TABLE OF CONTENTS

AUTHOR'S PREFACE

My wife Marilyn has been diagnosed with Alzheimer's disease (AD). Writing about it has helped me to cope and better understand her needs as well as identifying my needs as a caregiver. At times I feel so alone, so helpless and hopeless. I have found that writing helps me from emotionally exploding. The job of caretaker is a hard one. I have a family that cares, but as it should, the care responsibility falls mostly on my shoulders. I am frequently overwhelmed by repeated questions and frequent interruptions based on her needy concerns. I find myself needing a "time out," but then feel guilty about trying to escape the responsibility, even for a few hours. My walk is shared with my God, for as you will learn, my faith is one thing that has helped sustain me, but sometimes I find my soul screaming, "Where are you?"

Writing may be an escape; a respite from the daily battle with my acceptance that the disease is progressing, and that gradually each day may be worse. I may be writing because I need a catharsis—a chance to vent my feelings, expose hidden emotions, so that I can maintain my sanity.

I also recognize that my reasons for writing may be a little self-serving. By sharing my struggles, my light moments, my unending love, I may be seeking personal recognition for a job well done, some sort of kudos for me?

But I'm also writing in hope that by sharing my insights, my highs and lows, and my commitment to caring for Marilyn to the best of my ability, so that what I've learned may help others in their personal struggles. Over time, I have made a few notes about dealing with the disease. It occurred to me that my experiences might be helpful to others embarking on this painful journey. Thus this book was born.

As we learn about dementias we need to broaden our terms in order to understand the disease. Alzheimer's Dementia [AD] is only one type. There are other forms of dementia. What is common about them are care needs and the reliance upon caregivers, whether they be a care partner, or professional caregiving help. My experience is caring for Marilyn and her dementia. Other forms of dementia are vascular, Parkinson's disease, ALS, Huntington's disease, and stroke, to name a few.

Hopefully anyone caring for a critically ill person unable to care for themselves will find this book helpful. I trust that my insights will give you, the reader, the tools needed to help you and the loved one for whom you care. For those needing more information about neurological diseases, medications, care facilities and end of life care, you should first consult your physician. The references I have included and the classes provided by care agencies and the Alzheimer's Association have been helpful to me and I encourage you to seek further information to fit your needs. I do not pretend to have all the answers. I, like you, am discovering new sources of information as I read and learn from others.

As I share Marilyn's and my story you will find clues on how you too may survive the grip that dementia has upon lives. I have included in the final part of this book a Care Partner Survival Guide that I choose to call "Lifelines," an analogy on grasping a line tossed to you in a tumultuous sea to rescue you from the chaos and threat of drowning.

As with most of you who will read this book, some days are better than others and some days are really bad. The emotional overload is ever-present. There is always the umbrella of frustration of not being able to stop the disease. As you read on, you will learn that there is "light at the end of the tunnel" of memory loss. The light comes from the support one gets from professional support groups, as well as the light from your team of friends who share your needs. Essential is the continuing love and care that your family provides. The load you assume is too big to carry alone.

In this book I openly describe my successes, sorrows, and failures. You can follow me through discovery, learning about the disease, accepting the reality of the disease, and my saga of coping. I emphasize the importance of love, commitment to each other, hope, and faith. I get much of my strength from religious faith—in my case, a Christian faith. If you do not share my personal beliefs, please don't be deterred. The message is the same, no matter how you gain spiritual strength, whether from Judaism, Buddhism, Hinduism, Islam or any other faith that believes in a higher power. Regardless of belief, our needs are the same.

—Roger E. Riley
Newport Beach, CA

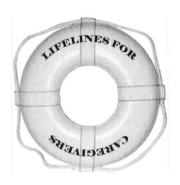

CHAPTER 1
NOW AND FOREVER

Who would have guessed that a brief glance through a shelf stacked with glasses, on a soda fountain counter at Curries Ice Cream store on the USC campus, would lead to love at first sight and a lifetime commitment of two people to each other! Marilyn didn't know it yet; she didn't even know me. It was my fraternity brother Ray Bartee who knew her. When I asked, he gave me her name and that launched my pursuit to know her. As I write this, we have recently celebrated our 59th wedding anniversary and look forward to our 60th.

Our years have not been all blissful. There have been some bumps on our road, yet our commitment to each other has been the glue, our respect for each other has been the fabric, and our faith has been our inspiration. On the inside of our wedding rings is engraved "Now and Forever" to remind us of our unfailing love.

We married very young, Marilyn 20, me 22, and both of us still students at the University of Southern California. I was going into my junior year of dental school; Marilyn had just finished her junior year with a MA degree in sight.

The first bump we encountered was the bump in Marilyn's tummy. We hadn't planned to start parenthood on our honeymoon. We certainly weren't ready to have children when barely out of the cradle ourselves. Thinking back, learning how to take things in stride and learning how to adapt has been our lifestyle.

Surprise: we learned that we were having twins! Kathy and Cameron arrived in the spring before my senior year. I had more than a year left before graduation. Tightening our belts, we moved to a larger apartment in a less expensive neighborhood. With the complications of a dual pregnancy, Marilyn dropped out of school and eventually had to quit her part-time job on campus as a secretary to the dean of the School of International Relations. To help bring food to our table, she laundered dental gowns for my classmates, competing with the local cleaners. I managed a part-time job collecting rental fees for my father-in-law's refrigeration business and had a weekend job driving a water truck and checking grade levels for my father's construction projects.

With family commitments, you might expect my career to suffer and my grades to go down. Quite the opposite! Up until this point, I was an average student mixing recreation, social, and beach life with my studies. I had yet to turn on the afterburners. With a wife and two children, it was time to really focus on my career. From being an average "B" student, I ended up graduating #4 in my graduating class of 105. Motivation is essential when a goal is in sight!

Marilyn and I moved to Newport Beach the afternoon of the day I completed my State Board Dental Exams. The exam was a dental operative procedure and had a time limit of 6 hours. I completed it in 3 hours, eagerly wanting to get on the road. We had rented a stake bed truck that was already loaded with everything we owned or had borrowed. Things were stacked high and dangling through the restraining stakes. Sort of brings back scenes from the *Grapes of Wrath,* doesn't it? As we arrived at our new home our neighbors, Barbara and Ridge Massey, greeted us. When looking over our truckload of stuff and crying children, they just shook their heads wondering what kind of neighbors were moving in across the street from them. They became our best friends, and over the years we continued to share the joys and sorrows of life with each other.

I had grown up in Burbank, California; Marilyn in View Park, a suburb of Los Angeles. I had spent weekends and summers in Newport Beach through high school and earned money varnishing and painting boats. Marilyn also loved Newport Beach, having spent some summer vacations there with her family. When we met, we had no idea we would make Newport our home. After marriage and planning a career, we both decided that this was the place we wanted to raise our children. The schools were great, and as the song goes, "the living was easy." This was the old Newport before high rises, shopping malls and mega-development.

Coming to Newport Beach was returning home for me. I am a 3rd generation Orange Countian and a 4th generation Californian. I was born in 1932 on my Grandfather's ranch in Tustin, California, where he was a tenant farmer growing lima beans on Irvine Company land. During the depression years, the only work my father could find was driving a tractor plowing the bean fields for his father-in-law. I was born in the farmhouse with my dad fetching the doctor in his Chevy and then kept busy boiling water and spreading newspapers on the dusty floor.

During WWII, the land was confiscated by the Army and turned into a "lighter than air" base with two huge blimp hangars. They were used as part of our coastal defense, to watch for submarines. The buildings are still standing—one directly over the site of the old green clapboard ranch house. I teasingly tell my grandchildren the blimp hangar is a monument to my birth. My early years were filled with many moves as Dad followed construction jobs to wherever work could be found. I grew up remembering stories while still an infant living in Red Mountain, a dusty roadside community on the way to Mammoth. We lived in a tiny trailer. While dad was working,

Mom stingily collected drops of water from a dripping faucet, saving money to do her laundry and cooking. Times were tough; work was tiring, yet from the stories I heard the community was close and the parties were fun and frequent. The family—Mom, Dad, my sister Bunny, me, and our cocker spaniel Susie—ended up in Burbank where we lived throughout my high school years.

Marilyn's life was quite different. Her parents also began as farmers. Her mother was from the small rural town of Banning, California and longed to be a city girl. Her Dad was a small refrigeration supplier in Los Angeles near USC. Marilyn's father sensed the future of electric refrigeration and became Los Angeles's first Frigidaire dealer. One of Marilyn's stories is about her Dad visiting Shirley Temple's home and designing refrigerator placement in Shirley's honeymoon cottage, which was a remodel of her childhood play house.

Marilyn was born in 1934 and was very special from the beginning. She was the third child, coveted and loved after her parents had lost her sister and then her brother to childhood diseases. They wanted everything for her and naturally were very protective. When it came time for high school, her parents decided to enroll her in a private girl's school. Marilyn balked; she didn't want to leave her public school friends, yet ultimately agreed to give it a try for a year. She later claimed that the school and all her many life-long friends was the best decision she could have made.

Our early married years were picture-book perfect. I worked hard meeting people, volunteering, getting involved in service clubs and most importantly, doing the best dentistry I was capable of doing. My training and skills began paying off. It seemed that we were the perfect family with a nice house, neat yard, clean car, a dog and a parakeet. We appeared to be what you could call a classic "All-American" family.

Once established, we welcomed into our family our third child, daughter Allyson.

Sure, we had some minor stuff—some marital bumps in our road. We were meant for each other but we also brought to the marriage two different personalities. I was outgoing, a gregarious, spontaneous, fun-loving personality, while Marilyn had a contemplative, thoughtful, quiet, personality. Yes, there were occasional fireworks!

Yet the commitment to each other we vowed on our wedding day, and the commitment of our love in nurturing our children, encouraged us through counseling to grow strong and overcome our differences. Our mutual respect and our faith smoothed out those bumps.

As a young mother Marilyn was perfectly happy to be a stay-at-home Mom. She got very involved with our children as a Brownie and later a Girl Scout leader. Our family camping experiences were a great training ground for overnight campouts with the girls. As Cameron was the twin brother with similar interests, Marilyn was also recruited to be a Den Mother for a Cub Scout gang of rambunctious boys. At Sunday school Marilyn helped out with teaching and snacks. In addition to all the children's busy activities she somehow found time to work as a Candy Striper at Hoag Hospital, with the National Service league volunteering at their thrift shop, as well being involved with the National Charity League.

Through our church activity Marilyn became a Deacon, until she had to resign from her duties as her workload of caring for our son became overwhelming.

The next bump in our lives turned out to be an almost insurmountable roadblock. Our son, Cameron, the most loving and needy child, the one easiest to befriend and the one needing the most hugs, was discovered to be learning-challenged. There were many years of psychological counseling and special educational experiences. The challenges became greater with an ultimate diagnosis of schizophrenia, with its accompanying violence, runaways, and deep bouts with voices and paranoia.

We loved him so much and wanted so much for him to be normal. Unfortunately, in spite of all our efforts, it was not to be.

While dealing with the trauma of our son's illness, there were signs of another problem emerging. Marilyn's memory lapses and other subtle indicators hinted at a more serious underlying problem. The "All American" family was about to face an even greater challenge.

As I confronted this latest setback, it was tempting to compare myself to Job. How many more burdens could anyone bear? Job laments: "If only my anguish could be weighed and all my misery be placed on the scales! It would surely outweigh the sand of the seas." [1]

This story is not about me, although it describes my journey from discovery to the present time and the challenges I faced along the way becoming a caregiver. My hope is that the support I've received and the experiences I describe will be of value to others who struggle with the challenges of being a caregiver for someone facing Alzheimer's disease or other debilitating diseases requiring a care partner.

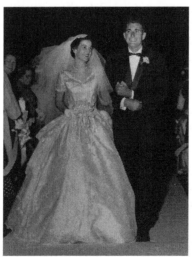

Roger and Marilyn, June 1955

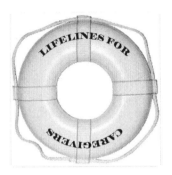

CHAPTER 2
DISCOVERY—THE EARLY STAGES

Our married life began as a typical Southern California family. We developed friendships from Junior Chamber of Commerce activities and an ever-growing community of friends from our local Presbyterian church, St. Andrew's. My professional career was going well. I was involved in community activities, and Marilyn was involved with her community service projects and many children's activities. Our lawn was mowed, there were no weeds in our garden and the cars were clean, even though the garage was frequently a mess from the many projects I was working on or from whatever boat I was re-building at that time. It seemed that we were an idyllic, "All-American" family, something like "The Walton's" or "Leave it to Beaver" of TV fame.

When we were in our twenties and thirties we had no suspicion of what the impact of Alzheimer's disease (AD) would have on our future. Our life was good and we were living happily, full of adventure and confident of the future.

In our forties, things changed dramatically and we began what would become twenty-five years of hell. It started with Cameron's illness and all the problems that accompanied it. This traumatic time certainly took its toll on me, and how much it affected Marilyn and his sisters one will never know. We are told that physical and emotional trauma systemically affects our body's ability to remain in a healthy state. While on this emotional roller coaster we definitely experienced unimaginable stress.

During this time Marilyn was treated for endometriosis with a hysterectomy and the endocrine imbalances that accompany these surgeries. The "All-American" family was experiencing some drastic changes to their idyllic lives and having to make some major adjustments.

At first, there were only a few signs of memory issues. Yes; there were the occasional missing keys. I attempted to solve that issue with a heavy brass key fob. There were some missed doctor's appointments—even a missed dinner invitation where, long after we were expected, we got the call, "Are you on your way?" Gradually I was noticing changes, but I was in denial that they were significant. However, they began happening too frequently to be ignored.

As the birthdays progressed into her fifties and sixties, Marilyn became less capable of organizing her time schedule, planning trips, and keeping up with the children's busy schedules. Many times she seemed humorous. She earned the nickname of "Gracie," after George Burn's wife Gracie Allen, for her off-the-wall, out of context remarks. Little did we realize this was a harbinger of her future struggle of knowing what day it was, mixing up the months, and not recalling what she had for dinner or with whom she'd dined. What was intended as a fun nickname instead became a cruel irony. Fortunately our friends and I realized this and quit being cute and began our commitment of support.

Marilyn's mother, a very organized, controlling person, began to fade in her seventies. She lost her ability to organize her home, to plan or cook a meal, or to find her way by car to familiar locations. She began to wander, and was once found on Pacific Coast Highway in Corona Del Mar wearing her nightie. We supported her and Marilyn's dad by providing occasional meals and spending time with them. My father-in-law was overwhelmed. He would shake his head and say, "she was just like her mother." Both Marilyn's mother and grandmother had Alzheimer's—though it was not called that at the time or even diagnosed. Yet, what we know today is that it was a disease similar to that with which Marilyn is struggling.

I began reading and studying about memory loss. Were the early hints something I should pay attention to? Was the disease preventable? Was there a genetic link? I had so many questions. I was learning about the disease and fitting some of the pieces into the puzzle.

In the Care Partner's Survival Guide *Lifelines* found at the end of this book I outline:

Common Warning Signs
- Memory loss.
- Difficulty in performing familiar tasks.
- Problems with language.
- Disorientation to time and place.
- Poor or decreased judgment.
- Problems with abstract thinking.
- Misplacing things.
- Changes in mood or behavior.
- Changes in personality.
- Loss of initiative.
- Difficulty in remembering recent events, names or appointments.
- Repeated conversations or questions.
- Confusion about current events.

Marilyn was experiencing many of the warning signs yet only in the mildest stages. If you were with her for a short visit or at a social event, her oncoming disease would be totally unnoticed.

I discussed my concerns with our family physician, Dr. John Storch. He listened attentively and assured me he had not yet noted any changes, yet bowed to my concerns and arranged for an evaluation at the University of California at Irvine [UCI]. In 2002 at UCI, tests were administered to evaluate cognitive decline. An MRI was taken to image the brain volume and a diagnosis was made. Marilyn had MCI—Mild Cognitive Impairment. Sadly, MCI often progresses to Alzheimer's Disease.

I can't over emphasize how important it is to find the right doctor. Most family doctors don't have the extra time or the extra training to recognize the changes. Here are some hints you can provide to help your doctor with his diagnosis.

Your loved one has:
- Begun to limit how much time they are around other people.
- Become sad or depressed or drawn into oneself.
- Stopped doing things that one has loved and done all their life.
- Become confused about the date and time of day.
- Become confused about daily and future events.

Memory loss is often not recognized initially, in part due to the preservation of social graces until later phases. Persons, not around the patient on a regular basis are usually unaware of the changes. You as the caregiver must help the doctor, your friends, and your family understand the changes. There are many standardized tests that are available for screening from your doctor. You may want to ask for a referral to a neurologist.

A frequently used test is the "Reisberg Global Deterioration" which screens for Alzheimer's-type dementia. Many hospitals have special programs to help you with a diagnosis and can give you advice on medications if they are indicated. In Orange County there is a program called "Vital

Aging" that administers tests free of charge and repeats the test yearly or bi-yearly to measure changes. Discussions with the UCI physicians and Dr. Storch were scheduled. It was early in the use of medications to ward off Alzheimer's. Aricept® was a brand new drug. I was informed of the potential side effects, yet did not want to deny Marilyn the chance of slowing down this dreadful disease.

Aricept® didn't help much and even degraded the quality of life with mood swings and depression. Clearly it was time for a change of medicine! After some changes to similar drugs, Namenda® was developed and it has been a godsend for us. Her disease has now plateaued and slowed to a gradual dementia increase.

Finding the right medications is not a one-size-fits-all approach. Staying on top of the medications available and adjusting her medication has worked somewhat for Marilyn.

The message I want to deliver is the importance of early diagnosis and appropriate treatment. We have dramatically slowed down the disease with the help of the medications. She has maintained her social skills, is always gorgeous, takes care of our home and expresses her appreciation for my weird meals. She never forgets to tell me how much she loves me.

She may not know what day it is, may forget to feed the puppy, or feed him twice, or be inconsistent in watering the flowers, but no matter. Though there has been progression of the loss of her reasoning skills and long-term memory, of the billion brain cells we each are given, 700 million are apparently still working perfectly for her.

I believe we have conquered this dreadful disease. You will find that I use the word *conquer* several times throughout these pages. Don't misconstrue it to mean that we have defeated the disease and it is no longer our enemy. Quite the opposite. What I mean to imply is that we have conquered the grip that the disease has on our lives. We have maintained some semblance of our lifestyle and preserved her quality of life for a prolonged time. With God's help, our lives will end from natural aging and Marilyn will not have to face the agony of advanced dementia with its loss of all recognition and shutting down of body functions.

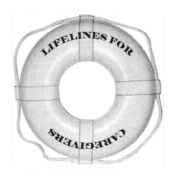

CHAPTER 3
LEARNING ABOUT THE DISEASE:
(YOU MUST LEARN, LEARN, LEARN!)

By learning about the disease you can conquer the consequences and not allow it to rule you. You'll be prepared for the changes. The disease is a moving target and each phase will require greater understanding. As you learn, you will find there is hope in its treatment. Learning will help you to accept, that, as of now, there is no cure or reversal. You'll learn to cherish the moments of joy and you'll learn to share your moments of agitation with your support team. As you share with whatever higher power you believe in, you will draw closer to your loved one as well.

Keep thinking: I can conquer this disease!

There are many resources. I'll describe the ones that have been meaningful to me. Also refer to the References at the end of the book.

Partnering with your Doctor.
Creating an open, ongoing relationship with your doctor is essential. Your doctor may be your family physician, an internist or a neurologist. They are the ones that will give the tests. You must communicate your observations and concerns.

They must rule out other physical disorders such as anemia, infection, kidney or liver disease, vitamin deficiencies, thyroid abnormalities, sleep disorders, and problems with hearing, blood vessels and lungs. All of these diseases may cause confused thinking and memory lapses. Your doctor may also give a "mini mental test" or refer you to an assessment expert. It is important to keep your doctor informed as you see him regularly, helping him with your observations of personality changes, eating habits, receptiveness, and time and date confusion.

Alzheimer's Associations
There are pamphlets, handouts and brochures that seem unlimited. They are a great resource in your quest of attempting to understand the causes and treatment of the many stages of Alzheimer's. One particular pamphlet "The Basics of Alzheimer's Disease" is a useful place to start. There are classes and workshops that can help you with crisis moments and estate planning. A meaningful class for me was a series that Marilyn and I both attended. We began with socialization exercises and then broke away into smaller caregiver and care receiver groups. In the small groups we were instructed about the methods of coping; a chance to grow together rather than grow apart. One of the most valuable services the Alzheimer's Associations provide is a hot line that you can call 24 hours day to help you through a crisis, or to refer you to one of their counselors. It is a ready source of information about:

- Alzheimer's disease and other types of memory loss dementia.
- Medications and other treatment options.
- General information about aging and brain health.
- Skills to provide quality care and to find the best care from professionals.
- Legal, financial and living arrangement decisions.

- The Hot line can be reached at 1.800.272.3900 or at www.alz.org.

The Alzheimer's Association also sponsors one-day workshops that teach the process of the disease, its stages, medications, and the role of the caregiver. These small group activities encourage participation and offer a chance to ask questions and to learn.[2]

Books

Still Alice by Lisa Genova, is a bestselling novel that helped me to look at the disease from the perspective of the person facing dementia—their fears and their need for acceptance. From my reading, I learned to be more empathetic. When the behavior becomes bizarre, when there is no recall and there is constant repetition, it is so important to remember it is the disease talking. Being empathetic humbles you and opens one's understanding, making your relationship with the one you love more whole and meaningful.

Playbook for Caregivers by Coach Frank Broyles is a great manual for caregivers. It is filled with sensible advice. Its organization makes a great game plan to follow. Use it to learn and to develop your own game plan.

The 36–Hour Day by Nancy Mace and Peter Rabins is another informative book. It has 560 pages crammed full of useful advice for caregivers. My early review provided me with information far beyond my previous readings. I look forward to having it as my bedtime manual as I continue to learn about the disease and how to prepare for the changes.

I recently read *What they Don't Tell You About Alzheimer's* by Robert Bernstein. Author Bernstein tells how he cared for his mother. He faced many problems with medical care, making decisions on professional care, and ultimately in preparing for her death. He went to extremes to care for his mother, even building a house nearby so he could take care of her. His story becomes very personal as you relate to his role as a care partner.

Films

I learned a great deal from the movie "Iris" starring actress Judy Dench. She portrays a high achieving, lively author with a love and verve for life, who begins to fade into the abyss of dementia. The angst and frustration of her caring husband, the collapse of his world, his health and his life style is so real, yet inspirational. It challenged me to live with the disease and conquer it, rather than let it destroy both of our lives.

The movie, "The Notebook" with Jim Garner as the patient, loving husband, sharing daily with his love, the beautiful story of their life and unfailing love for each other, challenges us to also share those moments with our loved ones. This film was part of my inspiration to write, to journal and even to write Marilyn's and my story so that we too can share these memories with each other and pass on our legacy to our children, grandchildren, and now great grandchildren.

Medications

The literature provided by drug manufacturers is useful. They describe the disease, the different stages, the use of drugs to moderate the progress of the dementia, and potential side effects. The descriptions of side effects and drug interaction are important to understand. A particularly well organized and useful booklet is "Caring for the Caregiver" published by Parke-Davis.

The National Institute on Aging, (www.nia.gov) has available booklets on pertinent subjects.

- Talking with your doctor.
- Caring for a person with Alzheimer's.
- End of life – Helping with comfort and care.

These booklets can be researched on line or can be ordered for your personal library.

Support Groups

Caregiving is a lonely occupation. You desperately want to share your needs with your loved one. However, as the illness gradually worsens there is grace in their unawareness of the grip the dementia has on them. They frequently are in denial of any changes in their lives and don't want to be needy or have special care. Most of the time you have feelings of being overwhelmed, unappreciated, and are unprepared to carry the load.

For this, there are the all-important support groups. I attended meetings of several different groups, including a men's group sponsored by the Alzheimer's Association, in an effort to find a group that best fit my needs. Ultimately, I helped found a group in our church. Because of the importance of this topic, see Chapter 9 for a discussion of support groups

Our caregivers group has been extremely meaningful for me in helping to learn how disease affects others; but more importantly, how others are coping and how we as a support community are reassured by the love we share for each other. Note that I used the word community, not a group of individuals but a community of support.

Be sure to include your friends and family in your support community. Loneliness is often a significant consequence for the one experiencing dementia, and also for the caregiver. The isolation we experience takes a toll on our health and quality of life. Humans do not do well in isolation. It is imperative that we maintain our personal connections with friends, church and activities. Old age is not a disease. We must learn how to age and accept its consequences. By maintaining our support community we can gracefully grow old together.

Finally, remember: It's our job to conquer this disease, for our loved ones and for ourselves. The grip it has on us is up to us!

Lifelines

Before writing this book I prepared a short compendium of essential information for caregivers that I use as a handout for support groups. I call this document *Lifelines.*[3] In it I've included an overview of the disease, outlined some treatment options, and summarized the most important actions that can be taken by caregivers, both to preserve their own health and to help their loved one who is suffering from AD. It is included at the end of the book as Chapter 18.

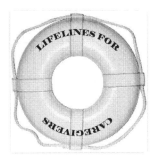

CHAPTER 4
ACCEPTANCE

Acceptance is one of the most difficult things to face. You will have to come to grips with acceptance that the disease is progressing, that your life will become increasingly chaotic, and you will be constantly reminded of your loss. It is not only difficult, it is contrary to your natural response, which is to fight back, deny the power of the disease, and to reverse the hold it has on you.

Acceptance requires giving in, not giving up!

You need to be prepared to accept what can't be changed, yet at the same time be willing to give the extra effort.

Two episodes in my life may have prepared me for the acceptance with which I am now struggling. They may seem disconnected, yet they stand out in my memory as moments that taught me acceptance.

One event I recall was on a sailboat race around Catalina Island. It was about 2:30 A.M in the morning and it was dead calm. Our sails were luffing, banging port to starboard with the rocking of the boat in a light swell. Our lead was disappearing as the lighter/smaller boats were ghosting by us. I was at the helm desperately attempting to maintain a heading, drifting in lazy circles. I was patiently searching for any wisp of a breeze and struggling to remain alert on the helm, when a frustrated voice echoed in the dark from a fellow crewman.

"Riley, you make me so mad! How can you be so calm? My reply to Peter was: "I made up my mind a long time ago. The only thing I can do about the wind is change my attitude about it." Acceptance is critical in learning to cope. It is not easy. You are constantly challenged. However, acceptance is part of conquering the grip the disease has on your life.

There was another learning moment when we were in the midst of caring for our son Cameron, as he struggled with schizophrenia. He had been in and out of care facilities and mental hospitals, had run away, and lived on the streets of San Francisco and San Diego for a while. In an attempt to get his life in order he spent some time in jail and at Joplin Boy's Ranch, a youth detention center.

We tried everything to help him: neuroleptic drugs, megavitamins, psychiatrists, and special schooling. When his violence was out of control, he spent time-outs in psychiatric hospitals and in juvenile hall. We even attempted the voodoo of demon exhortation.

All to no avail! His disease continued to grip his life. I was desperate. Cameron stole every moment of my time. My efforts to cure him were getting nowhere.

It was during this time that I too was losing control! I was expending huge amounts of time and energy and exorbitant amounts of money attempting to fix my son, my namesake and my bloodline. I was misled into thinking strength and knowledge should be sufficient.

I phoned a pastor friend of mine asking if I could visit to share my anxiety and desperation. He listened attentively— never interrupted as I cursed God for not listening to me and not helping me cure my son's disease. I was angry with God and I held back no punches. I had experience working on the docks and construction jobs, so I knew lots of vile words. In my anger and frustration, I let fly! I was very disrespectful. Don Maddox, my friend, put his arms around me and reassured me that in spite of Cam's behavior, in spite of my outrage, God was still in charge, loved me and had not forgotten me. Don told me that God forgave me for going it alone and forgave my sacrilege, but even more, he reassured me that if I had faith, God would support me through Cameron's and my crisis.

The encounter I had with my pastor made me realize the importance of faith and changed my life and my behavior. I no longer had to do it all alone. I could trust others to help me. I learned that no matter how I tried, there were some things I couldn't control. I was freed of that burden of hopelessness and despair.

From that moment I learned to turn my concerns over to God; to accept that Cam would be safe and I would be whole.

Cameron's disease continued in spite of the medications and supportive living he received. Our lives continued to be chaotic; yet from that moment on, I felt I had a partner to share my burden. Cameron no longer was my entire life. I was able to return to the joys of being a father and husband to the rest of my family. I was able to concentrate on my career. I was freed to live my life.

As his disease got further out of control, Marilyn and I struggled with acceptance of our situation. When Cameron was in the depths of his disease, on the streets of San Diego and San Francisco, I was treating him with tough love. If his life was to end I was ready to accept it as God's will. Marilyn, in contrast was begging me to drive to San Diego, find him and, rescue him. She, as always, was right. We found him and again tried our best to help him with counseling and medications.

I'd like to tell you that Cameron got well. He did not. My faith sustained me as we said goodbye to Cameron. The drugs that were helping him with his schizophrenia destroyed his ability to make white blood cells and he died from complications of a common cold, unable to fight off infection at age 39. As I held Cameron in my arms for the last time, I felt he was at peace, he knew he was loved, and that after twenty-five years of struggle he would be safe in the arms of God.

Even as I grieve the loss of my only son, his life and my acceptance, was possibly his last and most important gift to me. Learning how to take life's punches in stride was a valuable lesson I needed to learn to be able to face the insurmountable concerns of Marilyn's dementia and the changing roles that I would assume.

My acceptance of Marilyn's disease remains a challenge for me. I would like her to be a part of my busy, committed life. Sometimes I over-program our lives. On occasion I behave like a drill sergeant, barking orders to hurry up or in frustration trying to stop unnecessary or repeated questions. For her there are too many activities, too many people around. Acceptance to me may mean that her routines and slower pace may be more comforting to her; I may be the one who needs to change my pace.

As I have learned to share her needs with close family and friends, I try to bring them along, helping Marilyn and me with our needs for a personal support system. You will note that doing it alone is next to impossible. You have to develop your community of support.

Marilyn's cousin Stuart Schlegel, a retired Episcopal priest, shared his thoughts on acceptance and patience:

> "Without committed Christianity, I would not have been anything close to an effective caregiver for my wife. When she was deep into what I guess you would call 'The repetitive phase' she would say the same thing, or ask the same question over and over again. One day, after she had asked me again and again all morning whether she had taken a shower that morning, I decided just for the heck of it, to count how many more times that day she would ask the same

question. When we turned out the lights that night, she had asked the same question 46 more times. I tried to answer each one as though it were the first time, as indeed it was to her. Only God's grace, in the form of patience and compassion, made that possible. I only felt gratitude that I could be there for the love of my life."

Dealing with dementia seems more difficult than dealing with many other life threatening diseases. Cancer is certainly life threatening, yet has hope with chemo and radiation treatment of reversing and sometimes curing it. Stroke victims frequently retrain the damaged part of their brain to function. Heart disease can be managed with medication and surgery, returning victims to normal activities. This is not true with dementias. They just get worse with the passage of time. The only hope presently available is a slowing of the brain cell destruction. Our partnering role we share with our loved one demands that we accept that the disease will not go away. Our role is to be by their side as their brain slowly dies. To love, care and support.

We live in such an insecure society, attempting with cosmetics to smooth wrinkles away and brighten our smiles to unnatural brilliance. As we attempt to remain youthful, we sometimes miss the gentleness of aging—a time to accept who we are; a time to accept the highs and low blows of life; a time to let our love for our loved ones and our trust in our faith become a beacon showing us our way.

Have you ever stared deeply into the eyes of a dog or other beloved pet? What you see is love, loyalty, friendship, trust, and acceptance. Unconditional acceptance! Sometimes we need to take time to look in a mirror and to stare deeply into our own eyes. Are we capable of showing our love and care? Does it shine so clearly?

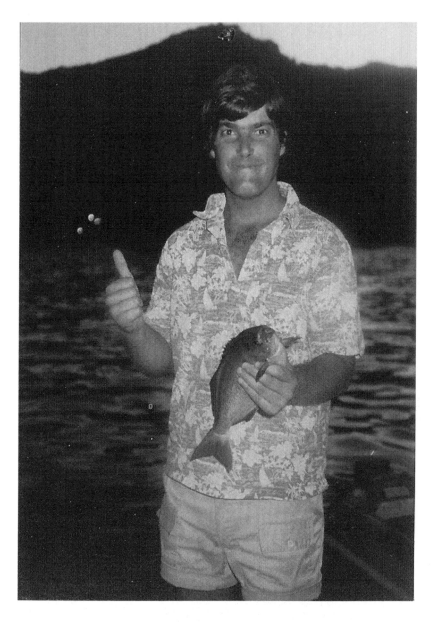

Cameron Riley, Catalina Island 1992

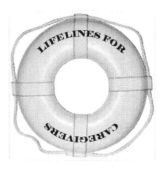

CHAPTER 5
MY FAITH—MY STRENGTH

A s you read this book you will note that I make frequent reference to faith and my belief in a higher power. This belief in my God has sustained me as I have struggled with the challenges fate has thrown at Marilyn and me, first with our son and then with her health. Yet, I recognize that not all AD caregivers can be believers like me because the disease itself is the ultimate agnostic when choosing its victims. Christians such as Marilyn are no more susceptible to AD than those who have never thought seriously about religion or simply choose to be secular. As caregivers, however, we all share the same need: a source for internal strength and emotional support that most often transcends that which we can reliably muster as individuals. If God is not your source as He is mine, some other form of spiritual support must be found to guide and sustain you through your most difficult journey.

Though Christ is now my Lord and Savior it wasn't always this way for me. I began searching for God early in my life. I was probably eight or nine years old. There was a tiny non-denominational neighborhood church five or six doors from my house. Occasionally I would dress up on a Sunday morning, no prodding from my mother, and attend the service by myself.

I was just curious; almost like something was missing. Mom and Dad never discussed religion. I don't remember a Bible in our home; certainly no one ever read one. I know my folks were godly, and if asked, they probably would have replied that they believed in God. Religion and faith to them was deeply personal, not something they discussed or displayed outwardly. I think you could say that their God was their good works. Unquestionably, they were hard working, moral, good citizens. Their ministry was about being exemplary people.

My curiosity about God and religious matters continued to nag at me. In junior high school my friends included a group of Mormon children. They were wholesome and had good moral values. In high school I was busy with water sports and an active social life and religion was not a priority. In college I recall once getting in a discussion on religion. I remember remarking, "Thank God there is a God—the weak people sure need him."

That statement pretty much characterizes me at that time. I was very self-reliant, cocksure and in control. I still had some curiosity about religion, but I didn't need a God in my life.

In my early thirties, that changed. Once Marilyn and I were married, we were busy with our children, school, and working part-time to pay the rent and keep food on the table. There just wasn't time for religion in our busy lives. Marilyn had grown up in an Episcopal Church but its ritual didn't appeal to me. After we moved to Newport Beach, a number of our new friends attended St. Andrew's Presbyterian Church. It was a local community church, with a very active congregation filled with young couples like us, and it had a reputable pre-school. When we joined St. Andrew's, it was to become part of the church community, rather than to find a spiritual home. Then trouble hit.

Marilyn was overwhelmed with parenting and I was working long hours at my job and involved in too many community activities outside of work and home. As a result, Marilyn and I gradually drifted apart. No longer were the differences in each other's personalities exciting. We argued and talked about separating.

Needless to say, I was devastated. How had I allowed this to happen? I prayed, for the first time recognizing that I needed help, that this was something I couldn't solve by myself. We sought counseling and somehow got back on track. This was a new beginning for me. Three years later I had the opportunity to meet Reverend Donn Moomaw at a couple's retreat at Forrest Home. This was an inspirational, watershed moment. I learned that God's kingdom was not just about good works. With Donn's guidance, I finally came to understand grace and my need to fully accept Jesus.

In the Preface to this book I mention my personal faith and encouraged you, the reader, should your beliefs be different than mine, to use your personal faith to look beyond your own strength and also seek your personal spiritual support from a higher power. To the skeptic, I say, what harm could it do? To anyone who has walked the path of caregiving, or is embarking on it, you will find the road is so difficult that you will welcome additional support and the ability to share some part of the burden with a higher authority.

I believe that God does hear our prayers. He answers us in subtle ways. He helps us with our short temperedness and forgives us when we lose control. He recognizes our anxieties and soothes us with his presence. He reassures us that we too must have a meaningful life and is there for us, helping us as caregivers to give willingly our care and love; and at the same time encouraging us to remain involved and healthy. It is so easy to wallow in the morass of self-pity and crushing responsibility, thinking, "If I can just get by this, then I can get on with my life." The truth is, our life is now! If we can't continue living positively, we face the very real prospect of becoming one of the **60%** of caregivers whose deaths occur *before* the very person they are caring for! As a minimum, you could find yourself joining the many caregivers whose quality of life, its experiences and friendships, are also shattered by the disease.

I encourage you the reader, whatever your religion, whatever your faith you adhere to, to call upon it for support and solace. And for those of you without some faith, do not fall into the trap of assuming you are strong enough to face this evil disease alone. While you may be capable of solely providing the care that is required for your loved one, you are not capable of doing the same for yourself. Help is available.

For me, I never forget this prayer:

"Lord: We confess our tendency to lapse into pride and self-sufficiency, rather than relying on you to equip us. As we share our faith, help us to acknowledge our weakness, in which your power is perfect."[4]

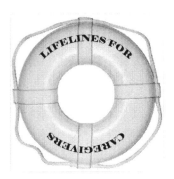

CHAPTER 6
THE ROLE OF MEDICATIONS

There are myriads of claims, scores of products: Gingko Biloba, Motrin, vitamin E, fish oil, coconut oil, the latest infomercial, and the infallible advice of the Ouija Board. Some may be of value, but most appear to be merely hopeful dreams for a cure that remains out of reach.

I admit to being intrigued by the claims because I want so badly for Marilyn to have her health and memory processes back. However, my scientific background encourages me to approach her medication needs with products that have been scientifically tested and medically approved.

As I stated earlier, Marilyn and I feel we have conquered the disease. She is not cured, for as yet there is no cure. But we have kept it from tearing our lives apart and in that there is victory. You will find that as a theme throughout this book. We are celebrating keeping Marilyn's memory processing dementia to the mild stages. It is now more than twelve years since her diagnosis in 2002. Most people with an Alzheimer's diagnosis are deceased or completely non-functional due to the progress of the disease 7 to 9 years after discovery. Marilyn's early diagnosis and discipline to her medication regimen has probably dramatically slowed the progress of her dementia.

In attempting to understand Alzheimer's disease, it is essential to understand that it is not about forgetting. It is not loss of memory, even though frequently misstated as such. In Alzheimer's, cellular changes occur in the frontal lobes of the brain, destroying the neurotransmitters; the cells that receive new information. As these cells are attacked, a substance known as amyloid plaque invades the brain cavity, progressively choking off the cell's ability to function. Some researchers believe the clogging of brain cells is due to dying off of cells choked from oxygen and may be related to low blood pressure or mini strokes. It is not until the later stages that patients lose long-term stored memory and cease recognizing family members and familiar objects.

I'm hesitant to share the medications we are using, since what seems to be working for her quite likely will be inappropriate for another. I am not a physician. You should consult your internist and neurologist as the best sources for medication advice in your particular situation.

As of this writing there are two approved classes of medications being utilized to slow the progress of the disease. The first classification is cholinesterase inhibitors, which work by slowing down activity that is breaking down the neurotransmitters. [5] Examples of these drugs are Aricept®, Razadyne®, Exelon®, and Cognex®.

The second classification of drugs help regulate the activity of glutamate, a chemical messenger involved in learning and memory. An example of this drug is Namenda®.

There are a few newer drugs currently undergoing research, searching for ways to dissolve the amyloid plaque. Some of these drugs have had significant side effects and are still under study. New drugs hopefully will reverse the effects of the clogged-up, dysfunctional brain cells.

In our personal voyage with medications, we were not immediately successful. Aricept® was the newest and best. Unfortunately it made Marilyn's quality of life worse, affecting her with mood swings, anxiety, and depression. After experimenting with other medicines in the same category, we decided to try the new category of drugs previously reserved for the most advanced cases. Her switch to Namenda® has apparently slowed the progress of the disease for the last twelve years.

As a trial, we added an Exelon® patch, a time release of cholinesterase drugs through dermal absorption. This combination of drugs is favored by many neurologists as currently the most effective. After several months I noted no improvement in cognitive function and recall, however, one of the side effects seemed to be an increase in antagonistic behavior. On the one hand she was standing up for herself. That's good! On the other hand, the confrontative behavior made my life tougher. We decided to drop Exelon and return to Namenda® alone.

As to off-the-shelf medications; she takes Motrin® daily to help keep the inflammatory process in control, Alpha Lipoaic Acid to assist neurological function, vitamin C, and a multiple vitamin. Her vital body functions are doing great. In fact, she takes fewer medicines than I do. At 79, her physiological age appears to be 10 to 15 years younger.

Research will continue to search for new drugs to help. Your primary physician needs to be aware of new medications and guide you in your needs. Many patients have multiple health needs. Some drugs can cause or increase confusion in elderly persons. These include:

- Antidepressant medications.
- Blood pressure medications.
- Heart medications.
- Narcotic pain killers.
- Anti-arthritic medications.

- Anti-Parkinson's medication.
- Tranquilizers.
- Barbiturates and other sleep medications.
- Restless leg and seizure medications.

Always let your doctor know of all medications you take. It never hurts to also consult with a trusted pharmacist. Since doctors tend to specialize and the drugs change so frequently, your doctor may not be familiar with some of your medications. Should you choose to do your own research, I find the Mayo Clinic, (www.mayoclinic.org) a useful web site.

Only recently have we been introduced to a very new experimental treatment that, with the use of low frequency magnetic waves, has the capacity to reorganize discordant and rogue brain activity. Knowing that Alzheimer's destroys brain cells—principally the frontal lobe—our hope is to improve that portion of the brain still functioning and help her with quality of life issues. After several weeks of treatment, her alpha waves, the brain waves that help us organize thoughts and actions, were significantly improved. There is currently a study being conducted at USC to determine if this treatment can be useful in Alzheimer's treatment. As of now this has not been accepted and is not covered by insurance. I have noted small changes in her expressions of happiness and organization. My hopes were for a miracle. The miracle may be the small changes and her improvement in her life quality. It is too early to tell.

Marilyn and I have volunteered for several studies done by a research center staffed by UCI neurologists. An early study that she was a part of was a blind study using a drug that hopefully would dissolve the amyloid plaque clogging her brain. That study was withdrawn due to complications of potential brain hemorrhaging. Fortunately we were just beginning and experienced no unwanted consequences. Both of us are currently in a study measuring cognitive function and changes in the spinal fluid to determine if chemical changes in the fluid may be a diagnostic indicator.

Another intriguing study that I am participating in is to determine if amyloid plaque can be found in the sclera of the eye and be an indication of early frontal lobe plaque formation and hopefully be used as an early diagnostic test. I fortunately can still pass the cognitive tests. In this study they needed persons as old as I, as well as persons who did not show signs of dementia. In every study you need a base line. This study is currently being done in the U.S. as well as in Australia.

Many people with AD experience what is known as "Sundowners." Patients experience increasing confusion as evening approaches. It is thought to be a disorganization of the circadian rhythm, much like jet lag. As in jet lag, some are being treated with melatonin, the natural endocrine produced by the pineal gland. This drug is available and many take it to regulate their sleep cycle, particularly when travelling through multiple time zones. The pineal gland, sometimes referred to as a third eye, is activated by sunlight and needs natural, outdoor light daily to replenish its hormone.

Most of these drugs and treatments can be very expensive. For those without means, good insurance is essential. You must also expect some large co-pays for many of the drugs.

Of course we hope for a breakthrough, something that will prevent the disease or bring about a dramatic reversal. We hope that science will have breakthroughs so that my daughters and grandchildren will not have to face the possibility that they too carry the genetic link, and if they do, will have more medical help for slowing or curing the disease. Lacking a major breakthrough, our goal is to delay the progress of the disease as long as possible.

The medications are only one way in which Marilyn and I have learned to conquer this debilitating disease. Staying socially active, keeping contact with friends and family, and other social activities are also important. Her social involvement may be as important in the slowing of her dementia, as are the medications. You will learn in the next chapter how we have remained involved with community, with friends, have learned to journal, to share our situation with others, and most importantly opened our hearts and lives to our faith, looking to it for help and guidance.

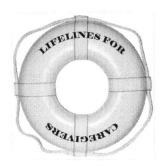

CHAPTER 7
IMPORTANCE OF SOCIAL ACTIVITIES

I can't over-emphasize how important it is to continue your social experiences. For example, if playing bridge is a favorite pastime, make sure your loved one continues this activity. There may be repeated conversations, there may be forgotten bids, however, the bridge skills remain. They are stored in the long-term memory bank and are still functioning.

Going out to dinners with friends is very important! Marilyn and I are very fortunate to have a group that refers to themselves as the "A Team." These are friends we have known for years, from church, from raising children, and newer friends we have bonded with from our boating club. We have traveled together, mourned the loss of companions, and frequently just get together for a meal and laughter. Most importantly, these are the friends that we can share our lives with, the ones who will be there when our needs become overwhelming. I personally have shared my concerns and needs more often with my A Team than with my daughters because I don't want to unnecessarily burden them.[6] They are my support team. How important it is for you to build your own support team? Very! Always remember, you can't do it ALONE.

We increasingly avoid large gatherings. It becomes more confusing for Marilyn, searching her brain for a familiar name or struggling to remember why she was there or whose event it was. There is always the fear of humiliation, of missing the point of a conversation or question. She looks so normal and to others around her she appears perfectly normal. In these times there are frequently old stories and events shared sometimes repeatedly, trying to retain her social skills.

Travel has been very meaningful for us. Planning has become more chaotic, since Marilyn has trouble putting together time, how far away it is, or whether we've been there before. Packing is challenging, since making decisions about what to take and remembering what has already been packed has become increasingly difficult. But when all that is behind us, there is the glory of travel. It is a chance to enjoy each other, to relax and be on a date with your very favorite person! Hawaii is Marilyn's favorite destination. When we go there, we experience some dazzling sunsets, some lazy mornings with papaya, granola and yogurt for breakfast, some delightful swims, sunning on pristine beaches, some nap time and a time for me to read, to write, and practice my art; but most of all a time to enjoy each other.

When traveling I enjoy journaling. I record the exciting and unusual events of the day and frequently will have a camera with me to capture special moments. Marilyn has always been the scrap-booker in our family. Those days are past. It is now my turn to help her remember our exciting moments. So, on each trip I take my notes and when at home, sit down in front of the computer and record our memories and download important photos, celebrating our fun-filled escapes. These albums are important for her and together we can recall our fun moments, and even more important, it helps me to keep focused on the joy that still remains in our chaotic life.

Besides the obvious value of rest and recreation, possibly the most important part is spending time with each other and making casual acquaintances. When we are traveling and meeting new friends we don't have to struggle to remember names and events. The conversations are always new and we are safe telling our favorite stories to someone who has never heard them before. It's a beautiful time to feel free and be who we are, a time to renew and refresh.

If you play the piano or the banjo; don't give it up. If you like to garden, don't give it up. Marilyn gets satisfaction ironing my many aloha shirts. Our ironing basket has never been so empty. This is her way of still being valued. As her reasoning and organizing skills have become more challenging, I have taken over the bill paying, cooking, and shopping. She remains involved in salads, table setting and all the thankless chores of cleaning up. Since shopping is one of my least favorite jobs, for meals we sometimes get by with unusual leftover surprises.

Don't forget games or puzzles. We have a favorite game, Rummy Tile, which always travels with us. I have 3 sets, one that I keep on our boat. Rummy Tile is like the rummy card game, where the goal is forming various number combinations. The difference is it is played with tiles like dominos. It is a very active and intellectually challenging. Marilyn and I have played it for years. It is presently beyond her ability to comprehend it. Yet, since she has retained her long-term skills, she is still very competitive. It is important to keep those brain cells active.

Outings don't have to be complicated or expensive. Take a scenic drive or a walk beside a stream. A walk on the beach watching the ceaseless action of the waves is relaxing. Many communities have evening concerts that are free. Make sure something that is dear to you becomes part of your caregiving fun. Look for things you can do together. With a spouse, dating is probably more important now than it was in your early romance. Plan to go out for lunch dates. Conversations are always best over a lunch table that you didn't prepare. Plan a night at the movies; a picnic at the beach or in a park enjoying a sunset. These moments preserve the youth in your love for each other.

Enjoy this time of your life when you are probably experiencing, like Marilyn and me, that never before have you been so much in love. It's so easy to feel unimportant and lonely when you are down. One's self-esteem is a valuable asset to maintain. Encourage your partner to dress up and go out. Sometimes she may need encouraging, or even special help in picking out a favorite outfit. Memory loss is frequently accompanied by loss of reasoning and organization skills. It is your job to be the fun planner since that is one of the skills she has probably lost.

I hope that each of you who read this book takes a good look at yourself in your mirror. I hope you see someone who not only has mastered the skills of a caregiver; but also has taken the time to cherish the joys of the past and nurtures the joy that still remains in your lives.

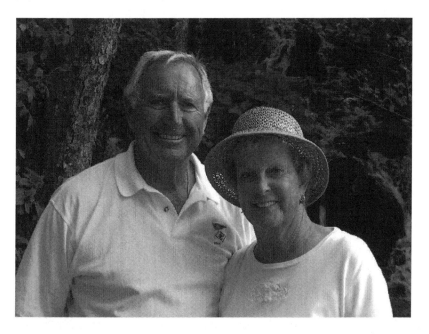

Marilyn and Roger 50th Anniversary

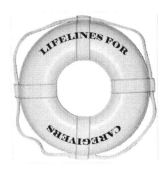

CHAPTER 8
SHARING WITH CHILDREN

I have always been the go-to guy. The nurturing by my parents rubbed off. I can do it; I will do it; I have done it. Not being in control is just not in my makeup. In our family I have always been the strong one, making most of the important decisions. I have also had the privilege to be "Captain Fun," the instigator of all the adventures we have been privileged to share with our children, their friends and our friends. It's been a great roller-coaster ride.

Now I am faced with needing to cry out for help, an admission that I am no longer "King Kong!" My knees are failing, I have chronic back pain, I have less energy due to ongoing atrial fibrillation, and to be honest, the birthdays are catching up. I can't decide which is worse, growing old or admitting to old age.

I would prefer to maintain the image that I'm still in control. I'd like my children, my close friends, and you the reader to think that, with all the positive advice I have and will give, that I have it all together, that I am above asking for help! Nothing could be further from the truth. I just don't want my needs to show. I don't want to appear as weak. This is also true about how I share the needs of Marilyn and me with our children. To them, I want to appear to be in control. I don't want them to be hurt by the pain of witnessing the progress of their mother's disease. I don't want to be seen as complaining about my role, my extra burden of caring for her. I don't want them to live in fear that they too might contact the disease. Their lives are very full and busy with their work, play, and family commitments. As a loving father I want to shield them from pain.

Telling our children about Marilyn's disease was difficult though I did my best to help them to understand. Shortly after her diagnosis, I gathered the girls, their husbands and the grandchildren and explained to them the mild stages of dementia, called Mild Cognitive Impairment (MCI) and the medication she was prescribed to slow its progress. I explained that MCI was a disease that impaired a person's ability to store new memory information. I said that things would be forgotten and things repeated. Yet, most importantly, no matter what changes we would be facing, Marilyn would always be Marilyn. Her love and care for them would never cease.

Reflecting back on that conversation, I recall not mentioning to the family what my needs were then or might be in the future. It was all about her needs. I guess I thought I was still self-sufficient, still the go-to guy

Several years ago I read Lisa Genova's book, *Still Alice*. There is an excellent passage within the book describing how Alice would like to be treated and remembered. I felt that her book would be very helpful to my girls, helping explain what Marilyn was going through. When Marilyn was seven years into the disease at age 73, I sent them the book, along with a letter that read in part:

> "I am giving you this book so that you may gain greater insight into what Mom is going through. Her experience is different than what Alice experienced.

Alice had early Alzheimer's and is portrayed as being much more aware of what was happening than is Mom.

"I'm thankful that you are so supportive of Mom and me and continue to care so much. Sometimes things are tough on us, sometimes I become overwhelmed and distraught, yet our love for each other and for our wonderful family carries us through.

"Mom carries the genotype that is most likely to result in Alzheimer's. This means that it is possible that either of you may also carry this gene. My prayer is that research will somehow discover a preventative or a cure for this dreadful disease, so that you or your children may not be affected. The genotyping is now available to you should you want to know if you are carrying this gene. This may even become more important as your children become parents.

"I know this is a heavy burden to bear. I love you so much; I need to share my fears. I respect you so much; I know you are capable of making your own decisions. I believe in you so much that I know that you too can be a survivor of this dreaded disease. Mom and I have not lost the battle. Our openness to the medication she has taken over the past seven years has smoothed out the disease and slowed its progress. With God's will, we can continue to live joyfully, madly in love with each other, sharing this dreadful disease together.

"I hope you will find this book useful to learn more about Alzheimer's. The title "*Still Alice*" brought me comfort as I realize that Mom is "Still Marilyn," even though some of her pages are blank.

"It is with much love that I share my thoughts. I love you both and pray that you can handle this gray cloud with love, patience, and optimism. Our choices are simple. We can let it get us down, or we can accept our fate and celebrate our lives and our loves.

"God Bless. Please keep Mom and me in your prayers as we keep you in ours."

I would like to tell you how well this worked in my need to share with my children. Quite the opposite! One daughter stated "Why did you send me this book? I read it and cried for days. I've never been so depressed.[7]

My other daughter has never commented. My feeling is that they prefer to deal with the potential of Alzheimer's in their own personal way. Meanwhile both remain physically active and asymptomatic. Hopefully new medications will be available for them should they have this dreaded gene.

In retrospect, I think the letter was more valuable to me than to the children. It was a way to share my fears and my needs. It was a way to share my love.

I'm slowly learning how to ask for help. I've learned to occasionally ask Marilyn's friends to pick her up for bridge. I occasionally will ask our daughters for help in packing, or closet straightening, or a shopping excursion. We are very fortunate that both live in California and are willing to help.

I recently arranged for some daytime companion help. I made a list of things that she and Marilyn can do together. This is a major step for me since I've been neglecting my own needs.

In my care-giving literature and in *Lifelines*, I repeatedly encourage you as caregivers to find time for yourselves to exercise, to socialize, and to recreate. I'm slowly learning to follow my own advice. I need to identify my needs, develop a workable game plan, share my needs with my support team, and learn to accept help. I pray for guidance and support.

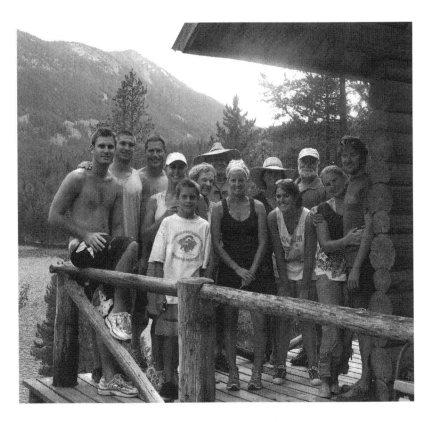

Riley Family in Montana

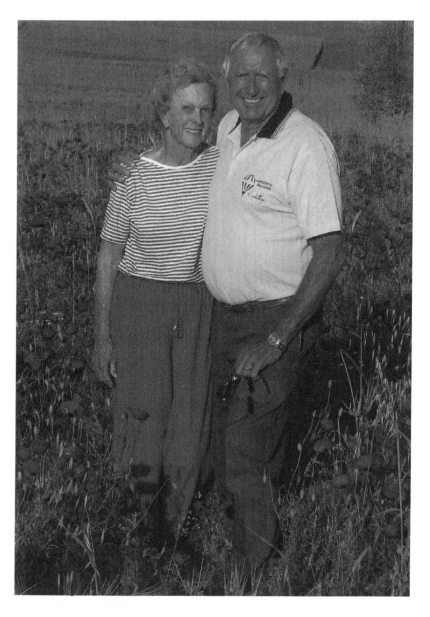

Marilyn and Roger, June 2009

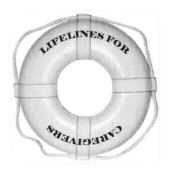

CHAPTER 9
IMPORTANCE OF SUPPORT GROUPS

Belonging to a support group has become essential for me and my fight with dementia. Since I am so involved, this should be the easiest chapter of all to write. Hopefully sharing these thoughts with you will lead you to find your own support group and receive the benefits it can bring to your life.

Marilyn and I attended a series of meetings sponsored by the Alzheimer's Association. One of the most important values I learned was to share my fears, my frustration, my needs, as others shared theirs. I lost my feeling of aloneness. There was magic in both the sharing and the support I was able to offer others.

I was not new to the power of sharing. As we faced our son Cameron's illness, I became active in a mental illness support group sponsored by my church and experienced firsthand how helpful was the power of sharing in helping others with their struggles. It not only helped each participant but at the same time helped me with knowledge of the disease and with my personal healing.

I attended a couple of AD support group meetings trying to regain the spirit of support I needed. Unfortunately, my early experience turned out to be "pity parties." This was not my style and did not meet my need. I was disappointed by the lack of spirituality at some of the groups. They were not sharing their burden with a higher authority, in my case, Jesus. They were all trying to do it alone—trying, by their own efforts, to overcome, to cope, to deal with frustrations, anxieties, and depression. The groups were about self-survival.

I then sought out an all-male group. This worked out better for me, yet something was still missing. The sessions consisted of each of us telling our story with some exchange of experiences. Each time it was the same story. There was no real process of study, learning, or discovery.

This led me to organize my thoughts. I had done a lot of reading, collected volumes of notes, and was experiencing a need to get my arms around this plethora of information. I took the approach of extracting and condensing the essential information and this became the origins of *Lifelines*. In addition to writing *Lifelines*, I proposed using the term "Care Partners" instead of "Caregivers," to better symbolize the partnership between the person receiving and the person giving care.

Lifelines became the springboard of my small group ministry, "Caring, Our Privilege Everyday" (COPE), a care partners support group at St. Andrew's Church.

I pleaded with the leadership at my church that a support group needed to be part of our ministry. I wanted a group to help me with my needs, and I was certain there were others who would benefit as well. I got polite agreement, but nothing happened. I shared *Lifelines* with the church leadership and nothing happened. It was time for action! Donna Shockley, my neighbor and a Deacon in the church, got together with me to talk about my idea. She also had a passion to serve this important ministry of our church. If we can believe the statistics, one in every five families worshiping at our church is experiencing some form of dementia within their families.

Donna and I signed up to take a facilitator's training course at Alzheimer's Association and became certified. As facilitators now well-prepared, we again approached the church leadership, this time with a plan ready for action. We got it: a room assignment and a notice in the church bulletin. We were off and running. We have met for the last three years. COPE is associated with the Orange County Alzheimer's Association. Our meetings are monthly for two hours. Within the group there is ample time to share our stories and share updates on our care efforts, our stumbles and our successes. We are a small group of 8 to 12 people gathered around tables. We respect each other's privacy and are careful to keep what we know and do within our small room. The magic in the room is the knowledge that we are not alone. There are others just like us who share our angst, our frustrations, our fears, and at the same moment share our hopes and our joy.

Donna and I work together keeping the group moving so each person has a chance to participate. She is always the quiet reminder to keep our spiritual house in order. At each meeting there is always an extra chair. It could possibly be waiting for you, but is always open for Jesus and symbolizes the presence of his spirit, bringing hope and rest to our souls.

It is my hope that you too may be inspired, not only to join a group, but be instrumental in forming a group to share your care partnering. Too often growing congregations are occupied with new growth activities. They forget about the needs of the aging population. If this group is missing in your church, stand up and be heard! Our needs are as important as pre-school or youth activities.

The COPE brochure (See end of Chapter) illustrates key points from our program. You can get additional details on our web site, www.sapres.org/support/cope. In the brochure we have attempted to offer information about Care Partnering in a condensed form. If you are a partner, or know someone who may benefit, you may find this information useful.

I'd like to emphasize: having one person ill is a tragedy; having two of you ill is a disaster. Don't be like I was, feeling I could go it alone. This point is brought home by an e-mail I received from a woman whose mother cares for her father.

"I want to thank you for the powerful ministry that you provide through COPE meetings. Since attending the meetings mother has gained emotional and spiritual strength and has grown in confidence and purpose. She is now engaged in life again and is thinking more clearly about the decisions that she faces.

Because of your support and encouragement she chose to spend Christmas in Solvang with my sister's family and we are planning another weekend away to see a film produced by my nephew. *She was previously homebound, feeling it was her responsibility to be at her husband's side.*

"Although the stress of her daily living has not changed, what has changed is that she knows that she is not alone and that there are other people in her same situation dealing with the same issues. She also understands that she must care for her own health and well-being and she has enough emotional energy and initiative to do this.

"Thank you for being there for her and for our family. We are grateful for your love and support."

I am grateful to this woman for summing up the value of a support group so beautifully. Sharing with others will be one of the most powerful tools you will have to help you conquer this dreadful disease and the grip it has on your life.

THE MESSAGE: YOU CAN'T DO THIS ALONE. DON'T TRY!

COPE—Support for Care Partners (part 1)

What is a Care Partner?

A Care Partner is anyone who provides help to another person in need, whether that's an ill spouse or partner, a disabled child, or an aging relative.

Caring for a loved one can be overwhelming!

Family Care Partners faced with overwhelming day to day tasks, often neglect their own physical and mental health needs.

Don't let it blunt your pursuit for:

- Social Interaction
- Work Responsibilities
- Personal Fitness
- Mental Health
- Sleep
- Recreation

You need not bear this burden alone!

COPE—Support for Care Partners (part 2)

Changing your family role is challenging!

As their disease progresses, your role will become more like a parent as your loved one becomes more like a child. You will increasingly assume family responsibilities and tasks they have always done.

Cooking | Shopping | Laundry | Finances

Taking care of yourself.

Family caregiving isn't just costly and time consuming. Studies show it could even harm your own health. Care Partners are at risk - 60% will die before their loved ones.

As a Care Partner, you may have feelings of:

- Sadness
- Anxiety
- Anger
- Depression
- Guilt
- Grief
- Frustration

These are normal feelings. It helps to share with others who may be going through similar circumstances.

COPE—Support for Care Partners (part 3)

Persons with memory loss are not the only ones requiring a loving Care Partner.

Chronic illnesses have similar care needs:
- Parkinson's
- Stroke
- Advancing Cancer
- Lewy Body Dementia
- Chronic Illness
- Physical Needs

Caregiving is a journey.

Families need help keeping their loved one safe and stimulated while managing difficult behaviors. The Care Partner's role is one of transforming one's self by:
- Learning and taking appropriate action
- Developing caregiving skills
- Opening oneself to the care of others
- Sharing one's burdens
- Looking to the Word for inspiration
- Trust and partner in the Lord's comforting embrace.

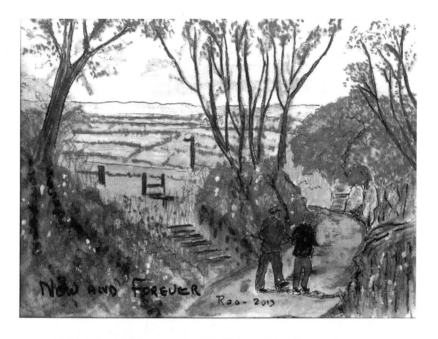

Now and Forever: Walking Life's Pathway

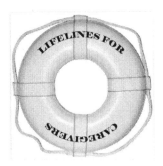

CHAPTER 10
MAINTAINING PERSONAL LIFE STYLE

Marilyn and I come from simple beginnings. Her parents were farmers and ran a small retail refrigeration business. My father and mother started as farmers and Dad went into construction as a grading contractor. Both sets of parents wanted their children to have a good education and were supportive of our college years. We have been privileged to have good educations and by hard work we earned success far beyond our parents' expectations.

As mentioned earlier, Marilyn and I are both graduates of the University of Southern California (USC). Thus it should be no surprise that football has been our fall passion since college days. As students, we loved the rooting section with the pom-poms and half-time card stunts. I even had an air horn confiscated from a large diesel truck, complete with air tank and air compressor. Yes, we were rah-rah USC fans. This enthusiasm carried over into our years at dental school and after graduation. When we moved to our new home, our neighbors across the street became our closest friends. They too were rah-rah USC fans. My friend Ridge Massey, though never a USC student, ardently adopted the team. This became a fall ritual: picnics complete with BBQ'S, tents, banners, and extravagant food. We are now celebrating over 50 years of USC fun. Our picnics are less frequent and far simpler. Some are just a sandwich enjoyed in chairs around an open tailgate. The memories are intact and the commitment to our school keeps us close. We share with each other the trials of our lives and the saga of our children. They are family.

The family football story continues. Our youngest daughter fell in love and married the USC football team quarterback. Needless to say when the guy we were cheering on the field became the guy who was to father our grandchildren, we enthusiastically followed him in his professional career, cheering on the Browns and the Cowboys when he played for them.

It seems that quarterbacks beget quarterbacks, so we've attended numerous football games including Junior All American teams, the Pop Warner league, and Newport Harbor High School games with our grandsons lighting up the end zone with perfect passes. How much fun to have someone to personally cheer for! Our youngest grandson is currently a quarterback for his high school team. We've got a whole lot of football left to enjoy.

Without doubt, our lives have been blessed. I worked hard while in school to earn my degree in dentistry. I've had a terrific career and was fortunate to earn a better than average financial return. Money has never been my goal; service for my patients has always been first. Isn't it amazing that when your priorities are in order; so many things fall into place? Our lives surely are blessed when we put our faith first, rather than ourselves.

I devoted time writing about football in our lives. I did it as an example of how we have preserved our passion for something that is dear to us. We may not dress as funny as we did when younger. We do not jump up and down as vigorously or as high. Our cheers may be a little gravel-throated, but we still cheer. We are able to preserve those memories. We are able to preserve those friendships. We are able to preserve our verve for living.

Living in a beach community, boating has always been an important part of our family life. Over the years we've had several boats, where we have entertained friends and families with numerous trips around Newport Bay and weekends at Catalina Island and along the California coast. We have special memories of Christmas Boat Parades and whale-porpoise scouting adventures with a group of underprivileged children from our community. The experiences have been priceless: adventure, great food, fun in the water and fun on shore with a barbecue and bocce ball games.

Since early childhood boating has been my passion, my hobby. I enjoy taking an older boat, fixing it up to my standards and maintaining it in Bristol condition. Marilyn and I continue to enjoy boating, even though now there are fewer guests, less packing and meal planning. Our trips are more spontaneous. Marilyn and I have found that quiet moments together are more meaningful. We don't need to be surrounded with activity as we once did. Sometimes just the two of us will escape to Catalina Island quietly enjoying simple meals, cozying up on the couch with a book or enjoying a sunset while anchored at Moonstone Cove. We also occasionally sneak away to our mooring in Newport Harbor, all of a mile from our front door, and spend a night or two on the boat, never leaving the harbor.

Travel remains important for us. We take trips to explore, trips to entertain or trips just to vegetate—to "kick back" and enjoy the love we have for each other. Our trips are simpler than many of those in the past. Air travel with artificial hips and pacemakers makes airport check-in chaotic. Packing becomes more of a challenge; and in spite of our effort, we still pack more than we need and frequently more than we wear.

Remaining involved in things we love is the stuff of which memories are made. We are still living in the present; not waiting until the knees feel better or medication improves the quality of our lives. Life is about living in the present, not about hopeful futures.

If you are physically unable to continue activities, you're never too old to revisit them in photos. If you are like us, there are stacks of photos that have never made it to the photo albums. Sit down with your loved ones and joyously recall your exciting romance and the joys you've experienced in life. This may be the last time to share quality time together—a chance and a time to celebrate this wonderful person! Those moments of joy and memory are still there in photos. Don't forget to name and date the events. As the years creep by, naming is important for recalling the wonderful times with each other.

One of our favorite escapes is packing a picnic basket and driving to Laguna Beach to a bluff top overlooking the Pacific. As the sun sets we eagerly look for the mystical green flash. Trust me! We have seen it and I even have it on film. My examples are not your examples. Yet, I suspect each of you has numerous memories and activities that you need to continue to celebrate. It may be a favorite campground, or a cabin on a lake. Possibly it is a family ranch house, a motor home trip or a cruise. You may get great pleasure from a drive in the countryside or a visit to a national park.

I also found that writing both Marilyn's and my life stories was a rewarding experience. If you choose to do this, your focus should be on the wonderful memories that you both shared together. Reflecting on happiness is encouraging, as we face stressful moments. For those of you facing someone's memory issues, memorialize their lives while you can still cherish with each other those priceless memories. With a loved parent; one of the most precious gifts is to sit down with them and review and record the priceless legacy they've given you. Your lives have been unique; take time to renew. I encourage you to take time to celebrate!

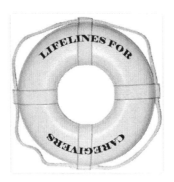

CHAPTER 11
MAINTAINING YOUR PHYSICAL AND MENTAL HEALTH

As the years creep up, maintaining physical health becomes more difficult. Frequently we are just too tired to exercise. Weight, heart conditions, arthritic knees, and collapsed disks seem to be part of the aging process. Just like our minds, our bodies need to continue to be stimulated, exercised, used! Don't forget the simple walk. Not only is it good for your muscle system and bones, it helps soothe your mind. It's a terrific thing to do with your loved one and if you have a dog to walk, everyone benefits.

Two years ago we rescued a six month old puppy, Meeko, a Havanese/Terrier mix looking for someone to love. It seemed the right time for Marilyn to have a companion. That turned out to be a good decision. He is something to love, hug and worry about. It's like a new favorite stuffed animal or a new baby to love. As Marilyn is losing purpose in her life, she has rediscovered purpose in caring for Meeko. If there is an empty spot in your life you may want to consider a pet. Meeko has truly added value to ours.

I walk daily with our dog. It would be better if I would also plan walks with Marilyn. Too often we are on different time schedules especially early in the morning. Not only is the exercise important, but regular exposure to daylight helps our glandular system regulate our melatonin levels and circadian rhythm helps with our sleep needs. For you, exercise may be tennis, golf, rowing or a vigorous game of bocce ball. What is important is that you still do something to keep in shape. Idleness is not only bad for the body as it accelerates muscle atrophy and weakness, it is also a form of brain atrophy.

I try to get to the gym 2 to 3 times per week. I have worked with a trainer to devise a series of exercises that won't aggravate my back and knees and allows me to work within the limitations of my cardiac disease. It's a short workout—by the standard of the young guys around me, almost no workout at all. It helps me keep my weight in control and also gives me a mental time out. I'm guilty of enjoying the shower more than the workout.

For your mental health, it's as important to remain involved as it is to keep exercising. Playing games, doing puzzles, reading for enjoyment, are all things you can do together. If you enjoy bridge, join a couples group or play at your local community center for seniors. There are centers like this in many communities. Take advantage of them. If it is a men's group at church make sure you get there regularly. If you are doing your own financial management, find a group with whom you can compare ideas. If you are fortunate and able to continue to work, even if only part-time, do it. I've been successful in rearranging things so I can continue to practice my dental profession one day a week. Being involved keeps me mentally stimulated and gives me a sense of worth as I help others improve their health and quality of life.

In your community there are places you can remain involved and gain a short respite from your care responsibilities. Many communities have a senior center with numerous activities. Some even offer short trips and cultural events. These centers provide a social environment as well as a place you can continue to be involved. How about an art class or a class to attempt to understand your computer? The YMCA may offer exercise classes and aerobic swimming classes. Many churches offer regular activities for seniors. The main message is there are ways you can remain involved with other people like you. As stated earlier and worth restating, idleness not only accelerates muscle weakness and muscle atrophy, it is suspected to accelerate brain atrophy. Watching television all day is not an option.

Don't pass up opportunities to get away with other groups of men or women. The stimulation of mini-retreats will send you home refreshed. I've had the great pleasure joining with twenty men from church for a ski retreat. I had never met most of them previously. I'm older than almost all of them. It was a chance for intergenerational bonding, an opportunity to make new friends, a time to worship together, and a time for renewal. I look forward to skiing with them again. Get out of your comfort zone!

A short respite, a time away from your hectic caregiving schedule, is essential. I have recently learned by my readings that a part of home care by professionals is also part of providing respite care for the care partner.

I have never been busier in my life, consumed daily with my care responsibilities, yet I have learned to escape to the creative side of my mind. I've only recently discovered how much I like to paint. When traveling, or on the boat, I carry a pack of colored pencils, a pad of paper and a water pen. The results aren't great works of art, yet I'm surprised how many of them I have kept and even framed. I've had no lessons and have little skill. I'm just letting loose the creativity that has been locked up inside me! This book is my first attempt at serious writing. In the past there has been the occasional lecture or a technical article, or most recently, *Lifelines*, the manual I wrote for caregivers. Personally, the most important thing I've written is *Voyages*, the life stories of Marilyn and me. It was privately printed for family members and close friends. I suggest, in your own way, let your own creativity bloom. I encourage you to also take time to record your own extraordinary life. If you try writing, focus on the joyful memories that you share with the person for whom you are caring.

In the Jewish tradition, it is a custom to write your legacy, and during your lifetime share it with your family. This is not your will. It is not about your assets. This is the legacy of your heritage, the legacy of your character, the legacy of your values. I believe, that as we experience memory lapses more frequently, it is our responsibility to consider the rich legacy we have to share with our loved ones.

Another Recommendation: don't put this off! There is no better time than now!

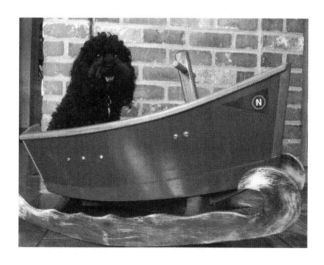

Meeko Takes a Boat Ride

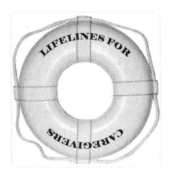

CHAPTER 12
KEEPING YOUR FINANCIAL HOUSE IN ORDER

Just as important as maintaining physical and mental health is to be a good steward of your financial resources. I know where I have stored most of my vital papers and records. I have written to my daughters so that they know the location of important documents. It's not all tied up in a neat bundle, however there is a trail—a paper trail that can be followed.

As for me, I have worked at getting my house in order. Marilyn is incapable of organizing all of the important data of death: the insurance, the home deed and mortgage, security portfolio, business sale, cars and boats, and so on. Should I precede Marilyn, it is my responsibility to provide information so my children can find the important records supporting my death needs as they also are overwhelmed with the need to support Mom. It's one of those things that needs to be done, yet is easy to put off.

Following is a checklist that may be helpful:

Plan for Tomorrow Today
Where is your will?
Does your family know where you keep your financial information?

Get Organized
The first step in getting your affairs in order is to gather all your important personal, financial and legal information and arrange it in a format that will benefit you now and your loved ones later. Then create lists of important information and instructions on how you want certain things handled when you die or if you become incapacitated.

Personal Information;
Contacts; friends, doctors, lawyer, accountant and broker.
Personal Documents: Marriage license, birth certificate, social security card.
Secured Places; Safe combo, security boxes and locked items.
Passwords.
Service Providers: Utilities, gardeners, cleaning service.
End of life wishes: Celebration and burial.

Legal Documents
Will: Location of original and attorney information.
Power of Attorney.
Advance directives.

Financial Records
Income and debts: Make a list of all sources of income. Do the same for any reoccurring debt.
Financial Accounts: List all banks and brokerage accounts, partnerships etc.

Company benefits: retirement plans and pensions.
Insurance: List all insurance including auto, RV, or boat.
Credit Cards: List all cards including card and PIN numbers.
Property: List real estate, vehicles and any other property you own and location of titles and deeds.
Taxes: Location of previous year's tax returns and contact information on tax preparer.

Insurance

You may want to consider long-term care insurance. The continued stress of being a caregiver could increase your risks of a heart attack or stroke. It is comforting to know that financial help is in place if needed.

Keep all your organized information and files in one convenient place, ideally in a fireproof filing cabinet or a bank safety deposit box. Review and update your information every year and remember to tell your loved ones where to find it.

Good luck! Remember, it's not fair to your loved ones to spend endless hours searching in all your hidey holes for your personal papers in the midst of grieving your loss.

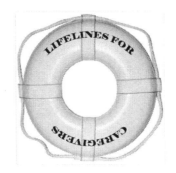

CHAPTER 13
HOW'S YOUR PRAYER LIFE?

This Chapter is a reminder, or a pep talk for me. Maybe it applies to you as well. As I've mentioned, I am guilty of attempting to "do it alone." I am hoodwinked by my strengths, knowledge, and wisdom into believing I'm self-sufficient! I've come to realize that I cannot do anything without the help of Jesus. In the Bible, Jesus says:

> "Come to me, all who are weary and burdened, and I will give you rest. Take my yoke upon you and learn from me, for I am gentle and humble in the heart, and you will find rest for your souls. For my yoke is easy and my burden is light"
>
> Matthew 11:28-30
> New International Version Bible

He doesn't make it very difficult. He says, "Come to me; I will give you rest." He doesn't say, "I will come to you." He says "Come to me." It is ours to ask. Each morning, when Marilyn asks again "What day is it?" Jesus says, "Come to me; talk to me; I will give you rest." Each day when I am overwhelmed by continual interruptions, questions and repeated questions over and over, he says, "Come to me."

These brief prayers help carry the burden. The prayers need not be complicated. It's an admission from us that the burden is too great for us to carry alone. I urge you to place your trust in your faith, where ever you get your spiritual strength, whatever belief it is that gives you comfort in knowing there is a supreme being that cares for you.

I find it very easy to pray for Marilyn, the children and grandchildren, the needy and the poor. The person I find it hard to pray for is me, the tough guy. I asked for help a number of years ago, when I was in the depths of caring for Cameron, our schizophrenic son. It was easy to pray for him. In hindsight, I was the one who needed the healing!

I had a session with Lydia Sarandan, a pastor and good friend at my church. She understood how hard it was for me to pray for my own needs. She wrote a special prayer for me. I'm better at this now than in the past and my needs are regularly included in my prayers.

If you need help praying for yourself, I encourage you to sit down and outline those special requests you have. Make your prayers specific. Don't just keep them rumbling around in your head. Write them down on a piece of paper. Take some time for reflective reading. Take time alone, a time to get connected with your needs, a time to share them with God.

As you pray try to immerse yourself in the confused thoughts of the one you are caring for, remembering their needs as well. Frank Broyle's book expresses their thoughts vividly with this poem from an anonymous author:

Poem

Do not ask me to remember.
Don't try to make me understand.
Let me rest and know you're with me.
Kiss my cheek and hold my hand.

I'm confused beyond your concept.
I am sad and sick and lost.
All I know is that I need you.
To be with you at all cost.

Do not lose your patience with me.
Do not curse or scold or cry.
I can't help the way I'm acting.
Can't be different 'though I try.

Just remember that I need you.
That the best of me is gone.
Please don't fail to stand beside me.
Love me "til my life is done.

                                        -Anonymous

CHAPTER 14
WHEN YOU'RE FEELING HELPLESS

I f the truth be known; I'm occasionally (maybe often) overwhelmed. In spite of my support groups and the other activities I've described in this book, there are times when my burden is overwhelming. I know I need a break on a regular basis. I've tried golf. Unfortunately my game is horrible, my back and my knee pain are aggravated; and what should be a great time away ends up being a rush to get through the game and return home to help Marilyn. At times I escape to the chores on the boat, my refuge and my comfort zone, only to hurry home to take care of Marilyn.

As I have explained earlier, I am not complaining about my care regime. Truthfully, I am possibly addicted to it. I thrive on preparing a good meal, managing our checking accounts, supervising the household chores and being the social planner. I admit that at times I resemble a drill sergeant, attempting to do everything efficiently

What I don't do is plan time for myself. I'm not yet prepared to turn over some of the care responsibilities to another responsible person. Could this be a feeling of guilt? By turning over some of the care, is this an admission that the disease is getting so bad that I can't handle it? Will Marilyn perceive that this means she is failing, her disease becoming more unmanageable? Will she feel that I have let her down or that I have given up? She has no understanding of the progress of her disease. She claims to be perfectly all right. She has no perception of my needs, but she is victim to my frustrations when I lose my patience, when my language becomes angry, when I cry out: Stop!! We've already talked about that!

A good friend of mine, Jack, was facing my same dilemma. He made the tough decision and employed a professional caregiver to come into his home two mornings a week. At first this did not work out. Jack's wife was uncooperative and resisted the intrusions into her home. Jack didn't give up. He persisted, and a second attempt with another caregiver was successful. By this measure he gained two mornings of escape to do things important to him. Others within my circle of support groups have also made this transition and express increased freedom to pursue their personal interests.

I am convinced that the quality of life of both the person needing care, and that of the caregiver, is much better off when they can remain in their own home surrounded by memories and the personal treasures acquired over a lifetime. It is my hope that Marilyn and I can be one of the couples that continue to enjoy that privilege. As of now, I'm still struggling with the problem that bringing in someone else to manage may not make my life more meaningful or lessen my burden. It seems that it may increase my load.

Let me tell you about a way I've found to "share my load." You may find it a little bit unconventional, but it really has helped me. A few years ago I went to a stationery store and bought a cheap spiral-bound notebook with a red cover. I call it my "Red Book."

It serves as a personal journal that has been valuable for me in crises. On the opening page I wrote:

Dear God, this life sucks. Following is a list of things I'd like to bitch about:

Then I would write down my latest concern, complaint, or worry. At the risk of shocking the reader, here is one of my recent entries:

Dear God; It's time to once more write 'my life sucks letter' and do a little bitching. You know how much pain and anxiety I am going through as I lose Marilyn. Her disease seems to be accelerating—more and more confusion, virtually no short-term memory, more dependence upon me. Her life seems to have an increasing loss of purpose and she has more personal awareness of her loss.

Yes, my concern is for her. However, she seems at most times to be unaware of how much she has lost. My concerns are also for me: I'm losing control as well; I've lost patience; I'm becoming forgetful as I try to be super-organized. I'm over-busy with all of my time consumed with her calendar planning, searching for misplaced objects, sorting out her confusion of events and her needy phone calls. She occupies my thoughts continually.

I'm not doing too well; my voice is tight; I'm constantly tired; my chest is tight; my belly is bloated; I'm anxious and on the edge constantly. I lose my control and temper, and when I feel overwhelmed, I drink more than I should.

I'm distracted from my project list. I reserve little time for myself and rush through those moments. When I'm away, Marilyn and her needs are always there.

I've lost the joy that characterizes me—the self you have given me. I need to change that.

At this point, I'm the one who's getting ill at an alarmingly rapid pace.

You know that I have attempted to cope through educating myself and writing and sharing with others the reality of the pressures and the burnout one experiences. Telling it and living it are two very different realities.

I've recognized the need for time away, which means someone to step in and help with Marilyn. As I struggle, I'm having a hard time defining what that is. I have been accused, by Marilyn, of doing things behind her back. It's true. I can't seem to tell her how worried I am for her and for me. I really need help, someone to be there for us. It should be someone to help with the decisions, not someone else for me to direct. Although it's premature, I probably need someone to live in to help with Marilyn and give me some time off.

I need to exercise more: gym, bike ride, walk, and yet I don't need to do this alone. I need guy time; some time on the boat, time at Catalina, time with the male side of the family.

Doing it all alone is adding to my struggle with depression.

God, help me to carve out the hours, help me to make a working schedule that gives time for Marilyn and makes time for me.

Help me with my prayer life.

Help me be open to your support and healing.

Help me as I struggle through the details of planning two lives.

Faithfully yours,
Roger

When I'm truthful, when I share my deepest fears, frustrations, and needs, when they are written down in my Red Book, a peace comes over me. I know God has heard me. I've gotten those pent-up feelings off my chest. Instead of looking to myself for answers, I am looking for help from Him.

As journaling has worked for me in the past, once I lay it all out, there comes a time for reflection and peace. A natural response is a flowing out of praise for all the good things in my life and my loving relationship with Marilyn.

It's magic!

From this deliberate effort of getting out of self to share my needs, to praise the good and positive, flows affirmation, the directions, the game plan that is directed by my faith in God.

In writing this chapter, I have disclosed my inability to come to rational decisions about my needs as I serve the needs of Marilyn. I continually anguish about getting help within our home. As of now Marilyn has resisted any attempts I've made to bring in a helping person. She is also very resistant to any mention of a day care facility. It is now my challenge to follow my own advice. Spell out my frustrations, my helplessness, my needs, and trust in my faith. **I will do it.**

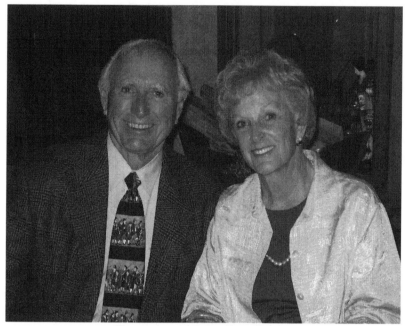

Roger and Marilyn 2010

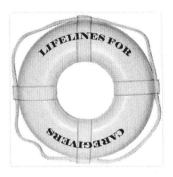

CHAPTER 15
MANAGED CARE

The subject of seeking managed care, assisted living, senior living, whatever you want to call it, is something we all resist. We all want to stay in our home, in our comfortable surroundings, for as long as possible. I am not capable of making that decision yet. Still, I am actively making my "Game Plan." From my readings I have learned that there comes a time when the care you provide in the home is no longer appropriate. At some point the home is inadequate for the needs of the care recipient and no longer fits the needs of you, the care partner. There are great sources of advice from care agencies and from the Alzheimer's' Association.

I have confessed to being overwhelmed and in the need of some help. I recently outlined Marilyn's increasing care needs and my subsequent needs to our physician at a regular check up. In this note I told him about Marilyn failing her driver's exam and my concerns about her getting lost even though her driving skills remained good. I explained that I was incapable of being the bad guy to the person with whom I shared my bed. He became the authority on both issues, explaining that he was recommending not driving and that we get someone to help me on a regular basis. Sometimes we need help in being the care partner rather the controlling spouse. Marilyn's cousin, Stuart Schlegel also was a caregiver for his wife. Here are his comments on remaining at home:

"Staying within your own home really seemed to me to be of great importance to whatever happiness Audrey was able to have. I am so glad that I was able to keep her home until her last month or so. But it got much, much worse. I had to accept that I just couldn't do it anymore. It was a hard thing for me to face up to, but I knew I had to put her into a nursing home."[8]

I realize that I too may have to make that decision for Marilyn and me. I need to prepare for that eventuality.

Another friend also made the difficult decision to place her mother in managed care. She had been caring for her mother within her own home for 15 months. She moved in with her mother after quitting her job and moving far away from her friends and social support. She, like many of us, is troubled about her commitment to her mother "promising to keep her within her own home." She wrote:

"So, as I live with my mother and observe her declining health, both mental and physical, I think about this stuff. I have reached a point that I no longer feel that I can care for her as well as she needs to be cared for. She has fallen in the night and cried out for me, like she cries out for me pointlessly all day; only this time it wasn't pointless. She was on the floor, had wet herself, gotten lost and confused between the nightstand, the dresser and the wall in the very same room she has slept in for 36 years.

"She needs educated decisions on medications. She needs someone to bathe her, dress her and help her eat without taking her frustrated insults personally. She needs someone with a strong enough back to get her off the floor or get comfy in bed. She needs someone who doesn't want to correct the distorted reality that she remembers.

"I need to put her in a home. I know that this is the right thing to do for both of us. She has gotten to the point where she needs 24 hour care. These days I work the 24-hour shifts and the lack of sleep has worn me down. Yet I feel like a slacker for wanting to do so.

"I'm torn. Should I let her finish her days in a home she no longer remembers because I said I would? Or do I write her name on her clothes in water-proof ink, pack her old Samsonite suitcase with her few needed belongings and move her into a home with strangers who will take good care of her?"[9]

This woman made the difficult decision that many of us are facing, or that many of us are fearful we will have to make. We know in our hearts that remaining in our homes, surrounded by friends and family and our precious memories would be our own choice. Her decision was made out of love for her mother and concern for the quality of her mother's care that she was no longer able to provide.

The key word is love; the compassion that your love is so great that you want the best for your loved one. When decisions about managed care need to be made, let the love you have be your guide. The job may be overwhelming, but never let convenience be your reason for seeking help.

This woman's mom experienced good care as she was moved from her home to a care facility. Her care partner felt renewed as she visited her mom, not merely to care for her, but now being able to cherish her as her Mother and to reflect on life's beautiful memories. When her mom passed away, joining her husband in heaven, the woman was able to say goodbye at her bedside, knowing she had done everything within her power to aid her mom.

Here is further information on this difficult situation from my readings of *The 36 hour Day*:

> "Like you, American families provide almost all of the care of frail elderly people. Seventy-five to eighty-five percent of all care comes from family members. Dementing illnesses cause particularly devastating burdens for family members. Because it is a disease of the mind, you are faced with the grief of losing companionship and communication. These diseases last many years, and caregivers usually cannot leave the impaired person alone for even a few minutes. Many caregivers are doing little more than surviving—just barely hanging on."[10]

You, like me, may need some time out. You'll need someone to stay with your loved one for part of a day, or a place where the cared-for person can stay for several days, or a nurse or caregiver to stay within your home so you can have a needed time out. This is known as respite care, because it gives you a break from caregiving. One needs to seek out family, friends and trusted caregivers to provide your loved one with a safe environment and you with a brief escape to reinvigorate yourself.

Another form of respite is adult day care. Many communities have programs that may be appropriate for you. The Alzheimer's Association is an excellent resource and can help you locate a facility in your area. Day care centers can provide:

> "...urgently needed respite for the caregiver and it often benefits the person with dementia. For most of us, the pressures of family life can be relieved by getting away

to be with friends or to be alone. The person with dementia does not have this opportunity. She must be with her caregiver day after day, but her impairment does not take away her need to have her own friends and time apart. The burden of this enforced togetherness may be difficult for the impaired person as well as for the caregiver."[11]

Be prepared for the person to reject care. Families often think their family member would never go to day care or accept a caregiver into their home.

"To the person with dementia, the new person in the house may seem like an intruder. The person entering day care may feel lost or abandoned. What the person says may reflect these feelings more than fact."[12]

"When you are already exhausted, arguments over respite care may seem overwhelming. You may feel guilty about forcing the person to do this so you can get a break. Make a commitment to yourself to give the program a good trial. Often the confused person will accept the new plan if only you can weather the storm."[13]

As a person caring for someone with a chronic illness you may experience feelings of sadness, discouragement, aloneness. You may feel angry, guilty, tired, or depressed. These feelings are appropriate and understandable. Sometimes it seems impossible to keep from being overwhelmed by your feelings. The re-occurring message in this book is to take care of yourself as you take care of your loved one. If you are having trouble being overwhelmed, please reread the Chapters on *Importance of Support Groups, Maintaining Personal Life*

Style, Maintaining Your Physical and Mental Health, and *How's Your Prayer Life?* When you're feeling helpless, when "go it alone" no longer suffices, my friend Jack Weiblen has offered some advice.

"While this situation most often arises when the loved one is well into the moderate to advanced dementia state, the care partner's advanced planning must begin sooner rather than later.

"Advanced planning is fundamentally giving consideration to the 'practical and financial impacts' of disease management options. Here is where the care partner's life really gets scary and complicated far beyond the daily grind of tending to a loved one. One's distress is heightened by complex intertwined issues:

- How fast is the disease progressing?
- What are the costs of various managed-care options?
- How do I financially prepare for what lies ahead?
- Will I be forced to sell or downsize our home?
- Are there accessible managed-care options in our community?
- Am I able to manage caregivers in an employee/contracting fashion?
- How do I cope when our "normal" social relationships pull away?

"Each decision-tree one experiences is unique and can become very complex, adding to the stress and depression associated with the situation faced. Where there are no easy answers and many similar questions, the process of working through the 'what if's' beforehand can provide some reassurance and hopefully mitigate 'crisis' decision-making at a time when reasoned judgment is hardest to reach. In my mind, attempting to honor what you believe your loved one would want, is only one of many considerations. It may not be the most important consideration."

Jack advises me to get beyond my "polyanna-ish plan of love, trust, commitment and prayer and face the practical truth that tough times may be coming and I, like you, will have to make some very tough decisions.

Coach Frank Broyles, in his book *Playbook for Caregivers*,[14] advises us to develop a personal Game Plan so that when the challenges crop up in your care plan, you are prepared to make those necessary changes with purpose, rather than panic. Each person's Game Plan will be different. What is important is that your plan not be forced upon you by lack of preparation. Seek advice from your family. Seek advice from your support team of friends. Seek help from the support group that I hope you have joined.

Should you need further reading I have included some helpful references in the bibliography that have been useful to me.

Make sure that your Game Plan fills your needs as well as the needs of your loved one. At all times remember that the game plan must always have the needs of the person you care for first, not what is most convenient for you, the care partner. Do this with faith and love.

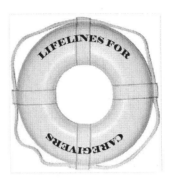

CHAPTER 16
WHEN MY LOVED ONE'S GONE—WHAT'S LEFT OF ME?

We all have had feelings throughout our lives: what would happen to me if Mom and Dad didn't come home? What would I do if the children didn't make it home from a date or make it through their illness? What would I do if my life mate ended up a casualty? Your deepest question: what would happen to me?

I, like you, have experienced these fears.

Would I become a loner? Would I run away and start a new life? Could I ever experience love again?

My life has been blessed by so much love, so much trust and so much compassion, and yes passion—that too. I feel that life would still go on. Marilyn would embrace the joy still within me. She would expect me to never forget the joys we had together.

Fortunately, we're not there yet! Our clocks have not run out. The time to celebrate our wonderful life is now. Our job as care partners has been reinforced by everything I have talked about in previous chapters. Never give up on dating your loved one. Surround yourselves with adventure and friends, talk about and make plans for your future with your loved one, find a support group you can share and grow with and never forget to include God in your sorrows and your joys. Ask God to hold your hand and guide you through the tumultuous times your future may hold.

When writing *Voyages* I felt it was important to muse about what life's end would look like. Marilyn and I discussed what our feelings about death were and specific wishes on what our burial and life celebration would be; but also on how we would choose to be remembered. You too should consider these important decisions.

I have had the privilege of being at the bedside of my father and mother as well as my son as I said my last goodbyes. In those quiet moments there was an outpouring of love and memories. Even as they apparently could no longer hear or talk there was the recognition expressed through their eyes of times well spent and love renewed. Never, never, fail to tell them how much you love them.

This book would be incomplete if it did not discuss the trauma of losing a loved one. Each of us will face death differently.

"People often have mixed feelings when the person they've been caring for dies. You may feel glad in some ways that the ill person's suffering and your responsibilities are over, but sad at the same time. There is no right way to feel after the death of someone with dementia. Some people have shed their tears long ago and feel mostly relief. Others are overwhelmed by grief.

"When much of your time and emotional energy was focused on the person's care, often for many years, you may find yourself at loose ends after the death. You may have lost touch with friends, given up your job or your hobbies. No longer carrying the responsibility you had for so long may bring feelings of both relief and sadness."[15]

I admit, my perception of caring for a loved one with Alzheimer's or other similar diseases that rob them of their ability to remember, or remain lucid in their final years may seem too much reliant upon faith and unrealistic expectations. Bernstein in his book expresses very clearly the dichotomy between faith and the reality of death in his Epilogue. He tells us there is no really good way to die; yet there are certainly bad ways to die.[16]

The reality of the anguish and traumatic circumstances are not in my game plan. Possibly, it may be time for me to take my own advice and learn from others as I re-read some of the great thoughts that are shared in the references.

For those of us that have maintained our support system of friends, family and a support group, the pain of losing a loved one will be easier. We will have people to share our pain and people to help us recover and plan our future. With faith in God, you will overcome even the death of a loved one.

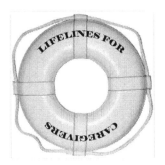

CHAPTER 17
EPILOGUE

Sadly, AD is growing problem, and it will only increase in magnitude with the increasing life expectancy and demographic increase in aging of populations. It is clear that it will affect more and more people, both directly, those that contact the disease, and indirectly, by its impact on those who care for those who are ill. Caregivers, or *care partners* as I prefer to think of them, are vital to the ongoing care and treatment of loved ones with AD or any other form of dementia.

Today there is a growing body of information available to help caregivers do their job. It is my earnest hope that this book can make a small contribution to knowledge for helping care partners do the best job possible and at the same time maintain their own health and sanity.

Hopefully you will learn, as I have, to cherish those unique moments that make your commitment to the one you care for special. It is easy to take on the burden of care in the manner of a drill sergeant attempting to maintain order amongst the chaos. This may not be the best scenario since it robs you of the joy of being that partner in their needy lives. Try not to shut out the joy of friends and family as you share your care needs.

My prayer for you is that you can look for and experience the joy that remains in your commitment to each other.

To date there is no cure for AD and the many other dementias requiring similar care. The most effective tools are early diagnosis, supportive medications and the loving care you may provide. With early diagnosis and prompt medical treatment, it is possible to slow the progress of AD and gain time for your loved one. This is important, as gaining breathing room for medical research to come up with new solutions may offer the hope of new and more effective medications and treatment options.

As of now, you, the Care Partner, *you* are the most important ingredient. To help you and all the others that will follow, I am donating all my proceeds from this book to the Alzheimer's Association and the important services they provide for support groups. Should you have the same passion, I encourage your support as well.

We'll all look forward to the day when AD is truly conquered.

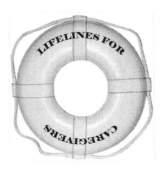

CHAPTER 18

Lifelines

A Caregiver's Guide to Survival
Understanding and Caring for Loved Ones with
Memory Loss

I have included *Lifelines* here in case the reader would like an outline on the needs of Caregivers. *Lifelines* is a compilation of thoughts gathered from many sources as well as from my personal involvement. I acknowledge in particular my debt to Frank Broyles *Playbook for Alzheimer's Caregivers,* which I found to be an invaluable resource. Here are the topics I cover in *Lifelines:*

Prologue: I am an Expert
I have lived through the stages of Alzheimer's Dementia (AD) with my mother-in-law and now for more than twelve years with the progressive AD of my loved one, my wife Marilyn.

I frequently am frustrated and agitated; at times I'm cranky and occasionally lose my temper. There are days when I suffer from depression and days of stomach cramps.

But I don't give up or give in!

I deal with my over-programmed life one day at a time, finding joy in remembering our past good times and excitedly planning our future.

I know that God has planned and equipped me to share the joy of caring and loving my wife, and this knowledge is sufficient to carry me through and to help me focus on what remains, instead of what we have lost.

Short Term Memory Loss

The frontal lobe of the brain stores recent memories. Short term memory loss starts during early stages of AD. The patient will not remember:

- What he or she had for lunch today.
- Who he or she talked to on the phone.
- What plans he or she has for tomorrow.

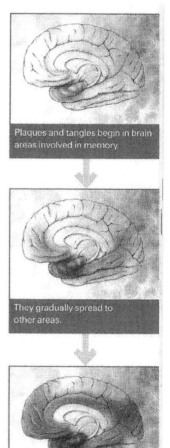

Plaques and tangles begin in brain areas involved in memory.

This is truly *not a loss of memory.* The information just did not get recorded in the brain due to disease-caused plaques and tangles forming and interfering with the storing of information.

They gradually spread to other areas.

Eventually much of the brain is affected.

*Illustrations courtesy of the Alzheimer's Association, "Basics of Alzheimer' Disease," pg. 11

Alzheimer's Disease Statistics[17]

Alzheimer's disease is a progressive degenerative disease of the brain. The cause is not understood and there is no known cure. It is the sixth top cause of death in the United States. The statistics are grim:

- 5 million disease victims today; by 2050 expect 14 million.
- Today there are 84,000 victims in Orange County, California where I live.
- One out of six people over 65 have AD.
- 50% of people over 85 have AD.
- 1 of every 10 persons and 1 in every 5 families are affected.
- The annual cost for AD care exceeds $100 billion.
- U. S. Medicare does not pay for long-term health care.
- Long-term health care insurance must be purchased *before* a diagnosis of AD.
- Lifetime cost of treating AD exceeds $200,000.
- AD costs American businesses $33 billion due to loss of productivity.

Leading Causes of Death in the U.S. (2010)*
1. Heart disease: 597,689
2. Cancer: 574,743
3. Chronic lower respiratory diseases: 138,080
4. Stroke (cerebrovascular diseases): 129,476
5. Accidents (unintentional injuries): 120,859
6. *Alzheimer's disease: 83,494*

*Source: Center for Disease Control

Stages of Alzheimer's Disease

AD is a slow, progressive illness. The easiest way to describe AD is in three stages; mild, moderate and severe. How quickly a person moves from stage to stage and what the symptoms are will vary from one person to another.

Stage 1: Mild AD

In the mild stage, the person may:

- Forget recent events.
- Begin to repeat the same thing over and over.
- Forget how to do simple tasks.
- Get lost easily, even in familiar places.
- Be unusually irritable or quiet.

Stage 1 usually lasts 2-5 years.

Many people do not see a doctor during this stage. It is important! The doctor may prescribe a medication that may slow down the damage to the brain. In my loved one's case, medications have kept the progress of the disease at the Stage 1 level for about 9 years.

Stage 2: Moderate AD

In the moderate stage, the person exhibits the symptoms of Stage 1 and in addition may:

- Pace back and forth.
- Have trouble recognizing family and friends.
- Neglect bathing and grooming.
- Have problems speaking and understanding.
- Become anxious, agitated, or suspicious.
- Have difficulty reading or writing.

This stage can last 2-10 years.

Stage 3: Severe AD

In the severe stage, the person may not be able to:

- Speak or understand words.
- Use muscles to walk or swallow.
- Control bladder or bowel functions.
- Recognize family or surroundings.

This stage may last 1-3 years.

AD IS NOT A CAUSE FOR SHAME! IT IS IMPORTANT TO KNOW THAT AD IS A DISEASE OF THE BRAIN, NOT A TYPE OF MENTAL ILLNESS.

Common Warning Signs

- Memory loss.
- Difficulty in performing familiar tasks.
- Problems with language.
- Disorientation to time and place.
- Poor or decreased judgment.
- Problems with abstract thinking.
- Misplacing things.
- Changes in mood or behavior.
- Changes in personality.
- Loss of initiative.
- Difficulty in remembering recent events, names or appointments.
- Repeated conversations or questions.
- Confusion about current events.

Coping with the Symptoms

It is important to know that the changes one is feeling may be due to the illness.

Some days may be better than others. The symptoms vary from one person to another. Not all symptoms may apply to each individual.

If your loved one stops doing things they have always done, such as bridge games, church groups, social contacts, etc., they may be worried that their friends will see that they are not their normal self.

They are aware in early AD that things are changing and avoidance and denial help them cope with their own fears and anguish.

Becoming the Caregiver

Changing your role in the family is tough. As AD progresses you may become more like a parent as your loved one becomes more like a child. You will find yourself slowly taking over the jobs they have always done, running errands, cooking, shopping, laundry, house maintenance, bill paying.

First Rule: Do not try to do this alone!

Set up times with family and friends, or church support groups to plan your day or weekend getaways. As the disease progresses you will already have a plan in place so that you can remain healthy and survive.

> **HAVING ONE PERSON ILL IS A TRAGEDY. HAVING BOTH PERSONS ILL IS A DISASTER! CAREGIVER BURNOUT IS COMMON.**

Finding a Doctor

Some family doctors don't have the extra training needed to recognize the changes. Early hints you can provide are that the patient has:

- Begun to limit how much they are around other people.
- Become sad or depressed or drawn into oneself.
- Stop doing things that one has loved and done all their life.
- Become confused about the date and time of day.
- Become confused about daily and future events.

Memory loss is often not recognized initially, in part due to the preservation of social graces until later phases. Persons, not around the patient on a regular basis, are usually unaware of the changes.

You as the caregiver must help your doctor, friends, and family understand the changes.

Remember: You Cannot Do it Alone!

Efficiency is doing things right,
Effectiveness is doing the right thing.
Peter Drucker

Take care of yourself! As a caregiver it is critical to recognize that you are at risk experiencing feelings of:

- Sadness
- Depression
- Stress and strain
- Anxiety
- Anger
- Guilt
- Grief
- Frustration

These are normal feelings. It helps to share these feelings with others whom you love and may be going through similar circumstances.[18]

To counter these feelings, develop your game plan!

- Put together your special team.
- Join a support group.
- Involve your family and friends.

You as the caregiver can't care for someone with AD and care for yourself at the same time. You don't need to. There are many people out there to help you.

Survival Tips[19]

- Put staying healthy at the top of your list.
- Have a backup plan in case something unexpected happens to you.
- Take one day at a time.
- Keep your sense of humor.
- Pat yourself on the back for the good job you are doing.
- Get enough rest and eat right.
- Make time for things you like to do.
- Talk about how you feel with others.
- Listen to your friends.
- Make a list of all the things your loved one can still do.

Daily Reminders

- Make time for yourself each day.
- Don't give up on the things you love to do.
- Exercise, eat right, and spend time with your friends.
- Share what is going on with family and friends. You need them and they want to support you.

Making Memories[20]

- Memory loss will get worse as AD progresses.
- It is now your job to become the memory.
- Spend time "dating." Go to movies, out to dinners, short walks, etc.
- Travel while your health still lets you.
- Create a memory scrap book or photo album.
- This may be the last time to share quality time together. A chance and time to celebrate this wonderful person.

Don't waste it!

TAKE TIME EACH DAY TO CELEBRATE POSITIVE THINGS!

Focus on what your loved one can still do, not on what they have lost!

Your Church or Caring Community: How can it help?

- Learn about AD and understand patient needs.
- Provide prayer support for patients and caregivers.
- Provide "time out" (respite care) for caregivers.
- Hold memory workshops.
- Offer useful activities, i.e.; preschool music and reading.
- Help prepare a list of things that can be done as a church and caring community.

Final thoughts: my best advice:

TREASURE EACH DAY AND LIVE IT TO THE FULLEST. CHERISH THE TIME YOU SPEND TOGETHER AND MOST IMPORTANT: LOVE EACH OTHER!

ACKNOWLEDGEMENTS AND CREDITS

I am grateful to the many people who assisted in the preparation of this book or who read the manuscript and gave me useful feedback and advice.

In particular, I thank my friend Pete Pallette, who introduced me to Craig Smith, my editor and publisher. Also, Pete's wife Harriet, who read my early notes and helped with grammar and punctuation.

My friend Ken Swift reviewed my first draft and made many helpful editorial comments. His comments in his second reading helped me to make this book more inclusive for others with a different sense of spirituality.

Jack Weiblen encouraged me and also was an excellent wordsmith for me in this book and the COPE brochure.

No book would be complete without thanking those many people who have inspired me to write. Special thanks to Ruth Lampe who introduced me to writing through a course she taught and for her editing and encouragement with this book. Thanks also to my wonderful support group in COPE for encouragement, especially Donna, Vicki, and Jack.

My special thanks to my beautiful wife, Marilyn, with whom I have had the privilege of sharing our wonderful life. We are more in love with each other today than when we were first married.

I'm grateful to Johns Hopkins University Press for permission to quote from Mace, Nancy L., M.A., and Peter V. Rabins, M.D., M.P.H. *The 36-Hour Day: A Family Guide to Caring for People Who Have Alzheimer Disease, Related Dementias, and Memory Loss.* Fifth Edition. pp. 179, 181, 182, 184. © 1981, 1991, 1999, 2006, 2011. The Johns Hopkins University Press.(Reprinted with permission of The Johns Hopkins University Press.)

I would also like to express my deep appreciation to coach Frank Broyles' family for permission to quote from *Coach Broyles Playbook for Alzheimer's Caregivers: A Practical Tips Guide.*

REFERENCES

Albom, Mitch. 1997. *Tuesdays With Morrie: An Old Man, a Young Man, and Life's Greatest Lesson.* New York: Broadway Books. Professor Morrie Schartz continues to give valuable lessons to a former student even as he lies dying of a terminal illness.

Anonymous. 1994. *Caring for the Caregiver: A Guide to Living with Alzheimer's Disease.* Morris Plains, NJ: Parke-Davis Co. A handbook for caregivers that covers understanding Alzheimer's, home care, legal issues and financial issues, and making home care safe.

Bach, Richard. 2006. *Jonathan Livingston Seagull.* New York: Scribner. Using the metaphor of a young seagull learning to fly, author Bach discusses the importance of seeking a higher purpose in life.

Bernstein, Robert B. G. 2012. *What They Don't Tell You About Alzheimer's.* Charleston, SC: Create Space. This is a memoir about a son taking care of his mother as she slips under the control of Alzheimer's disease. He details the onset of the disease and the gradual decline of his mother's health in an informative and sensitive manner.

Broyles, Frank. 2006. *Coach Broyles Playbook for Alzheimer's Caregivers: A Practical Tips Guide.* University of Arkansas Press. Frank Broyles assembled a team of experts to create a guide for Alzheimer caregivers. It is not a medical guide but has practical tips to assist in the care of a loved one.

Buford, Bob. 1997. *Half-Time: Changing Your Game Plan from Success to Significance.* Grand Rapids, Michigan: Zondevan Press. How to make the second half of your life more meaningful than the first by evaluating what you are good at and what you want to do.

Genova, Lisa. 2009. *Still Alice.* New York: Gallery Books: Fiction: The story of a fifty-year old Harvard professor's sudden onset of early Alzheimer's disease and how she and her family deal with her declining health.

Levinson, Daniel J. 1978. *The Seasons of a Man's Life.* New York: Ballantine Books. A description of adult male development, from mid-life to middle adulthood.

Mace, Nancy L. and Rabins, Peter V. 2007. *The 36-Hour Day: a Family Guide to Caring for People with Alzheimer Disease, Other Dementias, and Memory Loss in Later Life.* New York: Wellness Central, Hatchette Book Group. A comprehensive, 560 page guide that covers all aspects of caregiving, from evaluating initial symptoms of dementia to managed care.

Sparks, Nicolas. 2004. *The Notebook.* New York: Warner Books (Grand Central Publishing). In 1932 two teenagers fall in love. They meet again after 14 years in very changed circumstances. A notebook, read in a nursing home in the '90s, tells what happened.

U.S. Department of Health and Human Services, National Institutes of Health, National Institute on Aging. 2010. *Caring for a Person with Alzheimer's Disease: Your Easy-to-Use Guide from the National Institute on Aging,* Bethesda, MD. NIH Publication No. 09-6173. This comprehensive, 104-page handbook offers easy-to-understand information and advice for at-home caregivers of people with Alzheimer's disease. It addresses all aspects of care, from bathing and eating to visiting the doctor and getting respite care.

U.S. Department of Health and Human Services, National Institutes of Health, National Institute on Aging. 2008. *End of Life: Helping with Comfort and Care,* Bethesda, MD. NIH Publication No. 08-6036. This booklet describes care at the end of life, things to do after someone dies, and getting help for grief.

Other sources of information:

- Alzheimer's Family Services Centers
- Alzheimer's Association literature including brochures such as "Early-Onset Alzheimer's," "Behavior," and "Basics of Alzheimer's Disease." Also note the AD Hot line at 1.800.272.3900 and web site at alz.org.
- Prescription drug information. See *Aricept* and *Exelon* information regarding "living with Alzheimer's disease."

Film: *"Iris."* Actress Judy Dench plays a writer demonstrating the symptoms of Alzheimer's disease and progressing to advanced dementia. The devastation of her and her husband's quality of life and relationship are vividly portrayed.

J

Jesus, *27, 46, 47, 65*
Joplin Boy's ranch, *20*
journaling, *36*
Junior Chamber of Commerce, *7*

K

Kathy
daughter, twin to Cameron, *2*

L

legal documents
need to have organized, *62*
Lifelines
my guide for care givers, *v, vii,
9, 18, 42, 46, 59, 89, 110*
low frequency magnetic waves
new treatment, *32*

M

managed care, *75*
Marilyn
diagnosed with AD, vi
early signs of AD, *8*
student at USC, *1*
Meeko
our pet dog, *57*
Memory loss, *10, 38, 97, 100,
103*
Mild Cognitive Impairment
Marilyn diagnosed with, *10*
Moonstone Cove, Catalina, *55*

N

Namenda
AD medication, *31*
National Charity League, *5*
Newport Bay, *55*
Newport Harbor High School, *54*

P

physical health
importance of maintaining, *57*
prayer
importance of, *28, 41, 66, 72,
81, 87, 104*

R

Red Book
Roger's personal journal, *70*
Reisberg Global Deterioration
diagnostic test, *10*
rejecting care
may be an issue, *79*
respite care, *59, 78, 79, 104, 109*
Ridge Massey, *2*
Roger
early years, *3*

S

San Diego, *21*
San Francisco, *21*
social activities
games and puzzles, *37*
tpes of, *35*
St. Andrew's Presbyterian
Church, *26*
State Board Dental Exams, *2*
Still Alice
book by Lisa Genova, *15*
Stuart Schlegel, *22, 76, 110*
Sundowners
patient confusion at sundown,
33
support groups, *vii, 17, 18, 69,
70, 88, 99*
support team
importance of, *13, 35, 42, 81*
Survival tips, *102*

END NOTES

1 Job 6:1-3, New International Version Bible

2 Contact Alzheimer's Association at (800) 272.3900 or www.alz.org

3 Lifelines are the lines attached to life buoys and life rafts and the stainless steel cables that serve as rails on sailboats.

4 Thanks to Rick Kanwisher, 2014

5 Anon. March 2010: *Caring for a person with Alzheimer's Disease*, pp. 128-129, has a useful list of medicines used to treat AD and its symptoms, along with cautions regarding use.

6 My children have their own lives to live and families to consider. They are there for Marilyn and me in every way, but I try to spare them as much as possible.

7 Genova, Lisa. 2009. *Still Alice.*

8 Personal communication from Stuart Schlegel.

9 Personal communication, Blog written by a COPE participant.

10 Mace, Nancy L. 2007: *The 36 Hour Day* p 310

11 Ibid., p301

12 Ibid., p305

13 Ibid., p306

14 See Broyles, Frank: 2006

15 Mace, Nancy L. 2007: *The 36 Hour Day* pp 392-393

16 Bernstein, Robert B. G. 2012

17 Anon. 2010. *Basics of Alzheimer's Disease*, Alzheimer's Association, p 8

18 Broyles, F. 2006. p 13

19 Ibid., p 19 (repeated on pp 38 and 82)

20 Ibid.,, p 20

Made in the USA
San Bernardino, CA
01 December 2018